WOMEN'S PROBLEMS: AN A TO Z

DR VERNON COLEMAN is a Fellow of the Royal Society of Medicine. He is a regular contributor to both medical and popular newspapers and journals, and broadcasts frequently on television and radio. He is also the author of numerous books including *Guilt: Why it happens and how to overcome it* and *Stress and Your Stomach*, both published by Sheldon Press. He is married, with two children.

HEALTHCARE FOR WOMEN SERIES

HEALTHCARE FOR WOMEN

WOMEN'S PROBLEMS:
An A to Z

Dr Vernon Coleman

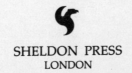

SHELDON PRESS
LONDON

First published in Great Britain in 1984 by
Sheldon Press, SPCK, Marylebone Road, London NW1 4DU

Note
This book is not intended as a substitute for the
medical advice of physicians. The reader should
consult a physician in all matters relating to health,
and particularly in respect of any symptoms that may
require diagnosis or medical attention. While the
advice and information here are believed to be true,
neither the author nor the publisher can accept any
legal responsibility or liability for any errors or
omissions that may be made.

British Library Cataloguing in Publication Data

Coleman, Vernon
  Women's problems.—(Healthcare for women)
  1. Generative organs, Female—Diseases
  I. Title   II. Series
  618.1   RG159

  ISBN 0–85969–409–7
  ISBN 0–85969–410–0 Pbk

Printed in Great Britain by
Richard Clay (The Chaucer Press) Ltd.
Bungay, Suffolk

PREFACE

'Trouble down below', 'a problem down there', 'a private matter', 'a personal problem' – the euphemisms are almost endless. And the fact that so many euphemisms exist illustrates very well the difficulty that many women have in talking about problems in and around their vaginas. They are often too shy or embarrassed to ask their doctors for help. The result is that problems which *could* be dealt with quickly, easily and effectively are left until they are difficult or even impossible to treat.

And yet it isn't difficult to get a good deal from your doctor when you've got a vaginal problem if you know what you can do, what you can expect and how you can use the facilities which are available. Understand your own anatomy, understand what can go wrong, understand what you can do to help yourself and understand when you must seek professional help and the benefits will be enormous.

To make the information in this book as accessible as possible I've chosen the simplest format there is: an A to Z directory of symptoms, diseases, techniques and technical terms. At the bottom of each entry there is a list of other related sections. Whether you're looking up a specific disease or a vague symptom you'll immediately find yourself being directed to those pages which contain the specific information you need.

Vernon Coleman 1984

WHEN YOU MUST SEE YOUR DOCTOR

1 If you are pregnant – or could be pregnant – and you have any problems at all.

2 If you have any severe pain.

3 If you have a pain that keeps coming back. Or a pain that isn't severe but which lasts for more than five days.

4 If you bleed between periods or after intercourse or your periods are heavier than usual. There are lots of harmless explanations for all these symptoms. But they can be an early sign of trouble. And the sooner you get help the easier it will be to clear it up.

5 If you have a discharge that is heavier or different to your usual discharge.

6 If you are worried.

ABORTION

There are two types of abortion: the spontaneous abortion (or miscarriage) and the elective abortion (or termination).

Spontaneous abortion

It now seems to be fairly generally agreed that one in every five pregnancies ends in a spontaneous abortion. If anything that figure is probably an underestimate since there are undoubtedly many women who abort without ever knowing that they were pregnant in the first place. The likelihood of a pregnancy ending in an abortion seems to increase with age and a 40-year-old woman seems to stand a forty per cent chance of having a spontaneous abortion.

In considerably more than half the cases where a pregnancy does end naturally the reason seems to be a problem with the foetus. There are many reasons why a baby may not develop properly and normally – the egg may have been old when fertilised, the mother may have had an infection or taken a drug – but the reason is usually a straightforward genetic fault. The fusion of an egg and a sperm doesn't always produce a healthy foetus and where there is a severe problem with the baby an abortion is usually the mother's body's way of dealing with the difficulty.

Where the fault doesn't lie with the foetus there are several possible explanations for a spontaneous abortion. There may be a hormone imbalance, the mother may be ill (with a generalised problem such as a fever, a kidney problem or diabetes), there may be a specific problem with the uterus (such as a congenital abnormality or a disorder such as fibroids) or there may be some nutritional deficiency affecting the mother and, therefore, the developing baby.

If a spontaneous abortion occurs after the twelfth week of a pregnancy then the cause may be some problem affecting the cervix, or neck of the womb. Two babies lost at this fairly late stage make

1

this a real possibility. If the cervix is weak or has been damaged in the past then it will simply fail to hold the baby in place. A gynaecologist can usually solve this particular problem by strengthening the cervix with a Shirodkar suture, which works like a duffle bag drawstring.

The danger that worries many young mothers-to-be, that of a baby being lost through an accident or trauma of some kind, is in practice a relatively rare cause of a spontaneous abortion. It usually has to be a severe injury or one specifically affecting the uterus to cause an abortion.

Nor are abortions usually a result of any past medical problem, of any previous abortion (spontaneous or elective) or of the mother having sexual intercourse during her pregnancy.

The first sign that a spontaneous abortion may be threatening is usually bleeding and the heavier the bleeding is, then the greater the risk of an abortion following. If there is pain as well as bleeding then the risk of abortion is higher. Again, the greater the pain then the greater the risk.

Since most spontaneous abortions are a result of a problem affecting either the baby or the mother (and usually the baby) there isn't much that can be done to halt the natural course of events. Indeed, since abortions usually start because there is a developmental problem affecting the foetus, trying to halt the abortion would be very unwise.

The only remedy most doctors recommend is bed rest, and to be perfectly honest, I doubt if this really makes very much difference. There is certainly no reason for a mother-to-be to feel guilty if she cannot rest and she subsequently loses her baby. If there is a real problem with either the baby or the mother then resting in bed isn't likely to have much effect. It is probably also wise to avoid sex during the time that the abortion is threatening (mainly because a woman who carries on having sex and then has an abortion is likely to worry afterwards that things might have been different 'if only …').

Once a woman has lost one baby there is no real increase in the likelihood of her losing another. But when a woman has lost two or more babies in early pregnancy then the chances of further pregnancies resulting in spontaneous abortions does go up slightly. She should certainly be investigated to see if there are any treatable causes.

After she has had a spontaneous abortion a woman should have a blood test to make sure that she is not anaemic. She should also wait three to six months before getting pregnant again – just to make sure that her body has a chance to recover properly.

Elective abortion

Pregnancies are not always welcome. If a woman is physically or mentally unable to cope with a child then she will usually be able to arrange to have the pregnancy terminated. Because of personal religious beliefs some doctors do not approve of abortion but a woman whose request for a termination is rejected by one doctor is quite entitled to seek advice elsewhere.

Obviously, if a pregnancy is to be terminated then the sooner the pregnancy is confirmed and the sooner the decision to terminate is made the safer the procedure will be. If an elective abortion can be done before a pregnancy reaches twelve weeks then most doctors will be happy to treat the woman as a 'day case' patient. In other words she won't have to stay overnight in hospital. Most doctors do, however, insist that when a woman is having an abortion as a 'day case' patient then she should be accompanied by a friend or relative, she should have no more than fifty miles to travel and she should make sure that her own family doctor knows about the operation and is willing to look after her in the unlikely event that any complications develop.

When a pregnancy has developed for more than twelve weeks then the chances of problems such as haemorrhage, infection and so on, interfering with the patient's smooth recovery are greatly increased. There is also a greater chance that the contents of the womb will not be entirely removed (producing an incomplete abortion) when the delay exceeds twelve or sixteen weeks. Although it is legal for pregnancies to be terminated at up to twenty-eight weeks most doctors are reluctant to perform elective abortions after twenty weeks.

The simplest form of abortion, performed within ten or twelve days of a missed period suggesting a pregnancy, consists of a menstrual aspiration – the straightforward removal of the contents of the womb. When the pregnancy has developed for more than a couple of weeks but less than twelve weeks most surgeons perform either a dilatation and curettage (in which the

3

inside of the womb is scraped clean) or a vacuum aspiration (also known as a suction curettage (in which the contents of the womb are sucked out with a device similar in principle to a vacuum cleaner).

When a pregnancy has progressed beyond twelve weeks the surgeon may choose to give the patient prostaglandins (which stimulate the womb to contract and thereby expel its contents), to inject a foreign solution, such as salt water, into the fluid surrounding the developing foetus or to perform a hysterotomy, in which the womb is cut open and the developing baby surgically removed. Very occasionally, if a woman is certain that she wants no more babies, a surgeon may perform a hysterectomy as a combined abortion and sterilisation.

When done by a trained gynaecologist in a proper nursing home or hospital an elective abortion is a very safe procedure. An abortion does not reduce a woman's chances of having a baby later and nor does it increase her chances of having a spontaneous abortion. Physical problems after an elective abortion carried out professionally are relatively rare. Mental problems are common only among women who have a strong religious background or who are exposed to propaganda produced by those who disapprove on religious grounds.

ACQUIRED IMMUNE DEFICIENCY SYNDROME (AIDS)

Although it usually affects men, AIDS has affected some women. The causative organism – if there is one – is still something of a mystery but the disease produces fever, malaise and swollen glands. The disease is a particularly damaging one since it destroys the body's immune system – leaving it prey to all sorts of infection. Sufferers contract infections because their bodies just don't have any natural forms of defence.

See also Sexually transmitted diseases (p. 74)

AMENORRHOEA

The complete absence of menstrual bleeding.

See also Period problems (p. 59)

ANAL INTERCOURSE

Some people (of both sexes) find anal intercourse extremely satisfying. And because there isn't much risk of conception they find it an excellent way to avoid the need for contraceptive use. The truth is that if it is comfortable and enjoyable then it isn't likely to do any harm.

There are said to be more bacteria in and around the average human mouth than there are in and around the average human anus so infection isn't likely to be too much of a problem. Sexually transmitted diseases can, however, be transmitted by anal intercourse.

Because the bacteria normally living in the mouth, the vagina and the anus vary, it is probably sensible to wash thoroughly before transferring attention from one sexual site to another.

ANAL PROBLEMS

Because the opening from the back passage (the anus) is very close to the vulva it is not always easy to differentiate between problems affecting the lower part of the gastro-intestinal tract and problems affecting the female reproductive organs.

When bleeding occurs, for example, it isn't always easy to tell just where the blood has come from. Is it inter-menstrual bleeding or bleeding from piles? When discharges develop it is sometimes difficult to be sure about their origins. Similarly it is often difficult to tell just where the pain is coming from. Pain in the rectum or pain around the anus itself can easily be confused with other varieties of pelvic pain.

As a general rule it is always wise to obtain professional advice about anything you're unsure about – particularly anything unusual. Persistent or recurrent pain, bleeding, discharge or any change in bowel habit – all these symptoms merit professional attention.

ANATOMY

The external, visible, sexual parts of a woman are known collectively as the vulva. The two outermost parts of the vulva are the labia majora, large fat-filled folds of skin which contain numerous sweat glands and hair follicles and which are normally covered in pubic hair. The labia majora are basically there for protection and their size, although it varies a good deal, is not of any real significance.

At the upper end of the vulva there is a pad of fat sitting on top of the pelvic bone. Known as the mons veneris or mount of Venus this fatty lump (which is, like the labia majora, covered in pubic hair) is there to act as a cushion during intercourse.

Just inside and roughly parallel to the labia majora are the labia minora, two delicate folds of skin which are usually free of pubic hair and which can vary in size quite a lot. The two labia minora aren't always the same size, by the way. The gap between these two inner lips is known as the vestibule and at the top of the vestibule the labia minora meet and go round the clitoris.

The clitoris is the female equivalent of the male penis and, like the penis, it gets filled with blood during sexual excitement. Not unnaturally that means that it gets bigger and harder. In some women this effect is best obtained when the end of the clitoris is stimulated; in others it is best obtained when the shaft is stimulated. Although the clitoris is sometimes stimulated naturally during intercourse it can also be stimulated by hand. Stimulation of the clitoris eventually leads to orgasm.

Still at the top end of the vestibule, and just below the clitoris, is the urethra, the opening which connects the bladder to the outside world. And directly below the urethra lies the vagina. It is important not to get these two openings mixed up for, if the urethra is mistakenly used in lieu of the vagina, incontinence and apparent infertility are two almost inevitable consequences.

This confusion can sometimes occur because in virgins the opening to the vagina may be more or less closed by a membrane called the hymen. Nowadays, this membrane is often split as a result of horse or bicycle riding or after the use of tampons but occasionally it is still there to be ruptured when a girl has intercourse for the first time. Some pain and a little bleeding often accompany the rupture of the membrane, remnants of which can be seen after as small tags along the inner edges of the labia minora.

The vagina itself is a strong muscular tube which stretches backwards and upwards from the vestibular opening. The walls of the vagina can stretch to accommodate a baby's head so there isn't usually any problem in their stretching to accommodate a penis. Just inside the vaginal opening there are two small glands (one on each side) which secrete fluid during sexual excitement and moisten the vaginal entrance. These are known as Bartholin's glands and occasionally they can become infected and swollen. In addition to these secretions the walls of the vagina also produce something called lactic acid which helps to kill off any bugs which might get inside an area which, being warm and moist, would otherwise be an excellent breeding ground for infections of all kinds.

The production of these secretions of lactic acid increases during a woman's reproductive years so that any risk of infection is kept to a minimum during the time when pregnancy might ensue. Before puberty and after the menopause the production of secretions drops away and soreness, dryness and infection are therefore common at these times.

Inside and at the top end of the vagina can be felt the cervix or neck of the womb. Also known as the uterus, the womb is usually described as hollow and pear shaped. It consists of extremely powerful muscles which can stretch to many times their normal size for months at a time. The lining of the uterus, the endometrium, is controlled by hormones and the bleeding which marks the end of each menstrual cycle is a result of the endometrium breaking down and being discharged from the uterus.

The womb lining develops each month in order to provide a settling place for any egg which might be fertilised and stand a chance of developing into a foetus. The eggs, produced by the two ovaries, get into the womb by travelling along two Fallopian tubes both of which open into the end of the uterus which is furthest away from the cervix.

If sperm manage to get through the cervix and into the uterus at roughly the same time as eggs are released by one or both ovaries then a fertilised egg may settle on to the prepared endometrium. If no egg gets fertilised, then the endometrium isn't then needed and is discharged ready for the whole cycle to begin again.

ARTIFICIAL INSEMINATION

For an egg to be fertilised a number of sperm have to get into the womb at the right time. Several things can go wrong and prevent conception taking place. If the ejaculate doesn't contain enough sperm, if the sperm are not active enough, or if the male ejaculates prematurely, there is unlikely to be a pregnancy.

These difficulties can sometimes be overcome by artificial insemination, in which the sperm are collected from the would-be father beforehand and then deliberately placed inside the would-be mother's womb at the time she is likely to ovulate.

Sometimes the problem is that the father-to-be cannot produce sperm at all or can only produce sperm of rather inferior quality. When this is the problem then one possible solution is to collected sperm from some other donor and to use that sperm to impregnate the would-be mother.

When artificial insemination is done in this way the donor usually remains anonymous. Lawyers still seem uncertain about the legal standing of any child produced with the aid of sperm from a donor.

See also Infertility (p. 44)

ASPIRATION CURETTAGE

Normally when a gynaecologist wants to take sample cells from the lining of the womb he will perform a D & C. Recently, however, a technique called 'aspiration curettage' has been developed. A long, thin syringe is poked in through the vagina, through the undilated cervix and into the uterus and a few cells are then sucked out for laboratory inspection.

8

Because the cervix doesn't have to be dilated this investigation doesn't involve an anaesthetic and doesn't involve a stay in hospital. It's all over in a matter of minutes, it produces nothing much worse than a period-type pain and it usually provides the surgeon with the information he needs.

See also D & C (p. 26)

BARTHOLIN'S GLANDS

Two small glands, situated just inside the vestibule, which secrete fluid to help lubricate the vagina. The fluid these glands produce make intercourse comfortable and enjoyable.

Occasionally these glands can become infected and swollen.

See also Anatomy (p. 6)

BIOPSY

Taking a small piece of tissue from an organ so that it can be examined in the laboratory.

BLEEDING

Whenever bleeding is a problem the first essential is to find out where the blood is coming from. There is a tendency to assume that any blood appearing in the vicinity of the vulva must have come from the vagina. In practice, however, blood in that area may have come from a local lesion of the vulva (a cut, laceration, scratch or tear), from the anal region (piles for example) or from the bladder and urethra (as may happen in an infection, for example).

When blood has been identified as coming from the vagina then there are a number of possible sources and explanations.

1 It may be a normal menstrual flow. In young girls who haven't yet started their periods the first bleed may be startling. Older women, who think they've passed through the menopause may also be surprised by an exceptional bleed. Women who have been pregnant and/or breast feeding may start bleeding again at any time. And, of course, there are some women whose menstrual bleeding is simply irregular.

2 The bleeding may be a direct consequence of pregnancy. At least one in five pregnancies end in spontaneous abortion and bleeding is almost invariably the first sign that something is happening. In ectopic pregnancies, bleeding may be a problem too. Finally, after a woman has delivered her baby bleeding may occur if the placenta or afterbirth hasn't been completely removed.

3 Bleeding may occur after intercourse. If a virgin with an intact hymen has intercourse there is commonly some bleeding afterwards. In some societies it is still considered an insult to the husband if a bride doesn't bleed on her wedding night. In most modern marriages, however, such an event is probably the exception rather than the rule. Bleeding may also occur after intercourse if a man is particularly rough and impatient. The vagina will normally lubricate itself and expand to accommodate even the largest of male organs but it needs time and preparation to do both. A woman who is frightened, nervous, embarrassed or unwilling will often remain dry and unrelaxed. In post-menopausal women the vagina's ability to lubricate itself diminishes and so bleeding can be a problem even if both partners are quite willing. Finally, bleeding may occur after intercourse if the cervix is any way damaged or inflamed.

4 Occasionally bleeding occurs at ovulation. This type of bleeding is usually very slight and it happens midway between a woman's two periods. It may be accompanied by a little pain.

5 Contraception is sometimes a cause of bleeding. The contraceptive pill occasionally causes exceptional bleeding during the first few monthly cycles while intra-uterine contraceptive devices (IUCDs) may also be responsible for heavy and irregular bleeding.

6 Finally, bleeding may be caused by straightforward physical problems such as fibroids or by unexplained hormonal abnormalities.

The solution obviously depends upon the cause. The only vital thing to remember about unexpected or irregular bleeding is that it must always be investigated. Cancer is a relatively rare but important cause of bleeding and is something that should be ruled out as soon as possible.

CANCER

For most people 'cancer' is probably the most frightening word in the dictionary. It has a dreadful public image. The truth is that although cancer is something that always needs to be taken seriously it can be controlled, it can be prevented, and it can be cured.

Cancer is often thought about and talked about as though it were some single, specific disease – like smallpox or tuberculosis. It isn't. There are literally scores of different types of cancer which affect human beings and these are often as different from one another as are the various different infectious diseases which exist. To say that someone is suffering from cancer is about as descriptive as saying that he is suffering from an infection.

Cancers develop when a cell or a group of cells in a specific piece of tissue suddenly change their identity. Instead of carrying on being bits of bone, breast, liver or muscle those cells may change their form and function quite dramatically. They grow, they multiply and they spread. They fail to do the job they were originally designed to do and they interfere with other cells around them.

Just why cells which were quite contented and efficient suddenly change in this way is still something of a mystery but researchers have found out that the change is often stimulated by some outside agent. So, for example, we know that there is a link between the smoking of cigarettes and the development of lung cancer.

The types of cancer which affect a woman's reproductive organs include: cancer of the cervix, the endometrium, the ovary, the vagina and the vulva.

Cancer of the cervix

One of the commonest cancers to affect women, cancer of the cervix (or cervical cancer) usually develops slowly and can often be completely cured.

For some years now researchers have been trying to find out just why some women develop cancer of the cervix while others remain healthy. After many surveys they have now concluded that cancer of the cervix is a special risk in the woman who started having intercourse at an early age, who has had many partners, who has had a pregnancy early in her life and who has had any sort of pelvic or venereal infection. Having sex during pregnancy seems to add to the risk since it appears that the cervix is particularly susceptible to damage at that time and therefore most likely to become cancerous.

The once popular theory linking cancer of the cervix to uncircumsised men now seems to have been discredited and most experts agree that it is the sexual activity of the woman, rather than the presence or absence of a male foreskin which decides whether or not a particular cervix is likely to become cancerous. That original theory about sex and circumcision was probably statistically sound simply because most Jewish women don't have sex during pregnancy or adolescence and tend to be less sexually adventurous as a group than their gentile sisters.

From what we know of cervical cancer there are three ways in which a woman can reduce her risk and protect herself.

First, she can remain a virgin for as long as possible and then remain faithful to one man. Becoming a nun would reduce the risk to an absolute minimum.

Second, she can use (or insist on her partner using) some form of mechanical contraception. By that I don't mean something fitted with clockwork but simply something that acts as a barrier between penis and cervix. Contraceptives such as the sheath help by preventing pregnancy (a risk factor) venereal disease (another risk factor) and the leaving of sperm in the vagina (some experts claim that it is seminal fluid which contributes to the risk).

Third, she can take advantage of the fact that cervical cancer tends to develop slowly and can often be picked up at a fairly early stage. With this end in view she should be on the look-out for any unexpected bleeding after intercourse or between her periods and she should visit a doctor or clinic for a cervical smear (see p. 18) at frequent intervals. Smears help because the cells on and around the cervix are fairly easy to obtain and examine under a microscope. If the cells look at all suspicious when examined in the laboratory then the appropriate preventative action can be taken. In addition to taking sample cells some gynaecologists also take a look at

12

the cervix too through a colposcope – a specially designed microscope which enables them to see inside the vagina.

Once a diagnosis of cervical cancer has been made the treatment will depend on the extent to which the cancer has developed. If the cancer is at a very early stage the gynaecologist may use cryotherapy, diathermy or laser treatment (freezing, heating or evaporating the cells). Alternatively the surgeon may remove the malignant section either by cutting away part of the cervix in a 'cone biopsy' or by removing the whole womb (a hysterectomy).

Cancer of the endometrium

Cancer which affects the lining of the uterus is more of a mystery than cancer which affects the cervix. Just what risk factors are involved we still don't know. From time to time it has been suggested that the contraceptive pill may be a problem, that a high dietary fat intake may be a cause, that leaving an intra-uterine contraceptive device in place for too long may produce cancerous changes and that the long-term use of oestrogen may be dangerous. All this is, however, still speculation.

Diagnosing cancer of the endometrium at an early stage is more difficult too since it is more difficult to scrape sample cells from the tissues and examine them under a microscope. This test is, however, now possible and will probably be used more widely in the future. Until then the most important thing any woman can do is watch out for – and report – any unexpected bleeding.

Once the diagnosis has been made the answer is usually to perform a hysterectomy.

Cancer of the ovary

Cancer of the ovary isn't as easy to diagnose as cancer of the cervix (mainly because the ovaries aren't as easy to see as the cervix) and may only be spotted when the ovary reaches an easily noticeable size. Sometimes the amount of swelling may be considerable and may be accompanied by a substantial amount of discomfort. To make the diagnosis firm the surgeon will usually need to look inside the abdomen and examine the ovaries and the tissues around them.

Once a diagnosis of ovarian cancer has been confirmed the treatment usually involves the surgical removal of both ovaries and the uterus. Both ovaries are usually removed, by the way, even if only one is obviously affected. The womb is removed too because, if the cancer has spread, that's the area most likely to be involved. Examination of the womb with the naked eye just won't show whether it is affected or not. Taking the uterus out improves the patient's chances and since the ovaries are going anyway, there isn't any question of the patient being denied possible future pregnancies.

Radium treatment and anti-cancer drugs are sometimes used in the treatment of patients who have had ovarian cancer and these therapies can be very effective.

Cancer of the vagina

Chronic irritation due to forgotten pessaries is said to cause half of all cases of vaginal cancer. It is also known that if a woman who takes diethylstilboestrol during pregnancy (it isn't prescribed these days) has a baby daughter then that child will grow up with a greater than average chance of developing vaginal cancer. Finally, it has also been suggested that some spermicides can cause vaginal cancer. The evidence against spermicides isn't universal or overwhelming but since it now seems that they are ineffective forms of contraception, and unnecessary when used in conjunction with other barrier methods of contraception, I don't think their status need worry us too much.

Cancer of the vagina is a relatively rare cancer but since it involves a fairly visible part of the body a regular self-examination will help to ensure that any problems are dealt with at an early stage. Look for retained tampons or other objects and check for any signs of bleeding.

Cancer of the vulva

Cancer of the vulva is rare and usually only affects women well past the menopause. It is thought that various sexually transmitted diseases may eventually produce cancer of the vulva. The early signs to look out for are ulcers, warts, lumps, discharges, irritation and bleeding. Any change which lasts for more than five days certainly needs examining by a doctor.

CANDIDA

Also known as thrush or vulvo–vaginitis, this is an extremely common infection. Thick white patches appear around the vulva and itching, soreness and pain on intercourse are common complaints.

The bug that causes the infection isn't anything particularly unusual. It lives on the skin of most people fairly routinely. It's only when the bugs multiply and take over that they cause problems, and although a candida infection can be a sexually transmitted disease (in that if a man has a candida infection on his penis he may pass enough extra bugs on to a woman for her to develop an overt infection too), the symptoms can develop without intercourse taking place at all.

The chances of a candida infection developing are increased when the naturally rather warm and moist area around and within the vulva becomes warmer and more moist (as can happen if nylon panties, tights, or close fitting jeans or trousers are worn), when there are changes in the amount of circulating oestrogen (as happens during pregnancy or when a woman takes the contraceptive pill), when the skin is broken (by scratches or abrasions produced by itching or by unusually enthusiastic love-making), when the amount of sugar in the body increases (as it does in diabetics), when antibiotics are taken (because they upset the natural balance of bugs in and around the vulval area) or when the whole area isn't kept as clean and fresh as possible.

Obesity makes candida more likely because it increases the chances of fatty folds around the groins keeping the vulva unusually moist and hot, inserting pessaries or tampons without washing the hands first can cause infection because candida bugs can affect the nails, and eating a carbohydrate-rich diet can increase the likelihood of a candida infection because it increases the body's sugar supply and thereby encourages the growth of the organisms.

Knowing how and why a candida infection develops, it is of course possible to do a great deal to help reduce the chances of contracting thrush. Good local hygiene is obviously important but it isn't necessary to use antiseptics or deodorants. Indeed, there is a real risk that using such products could increase the hazard by irritating the area. Skirts and stockings, cotton pants or no pants at all are better by far than nylon underwear, tights and jeans or trousers. (The largest single factor contributing to the current epidemic of candida has probably been the widespread popularity of tights and the demise of old-fashioned stockings. Written by a man, that sounds sexist but even women doctors agree with it!) Perfumed soaps should be avoided because they can irritate too and antibiotics should only ever be taken when they are really necessary. If you need to take an antibiotic and you do suffer from candida infections then it might be worthwhile using an antifungal cream or pessary at the same time.

Women who take the progestogen-only pill (as opposed to the combined pill) are less likely to get a candida infection and women whose partners use condoms are less likely than either group (seminal fluid is an excellent culture medium for candida).

Once a candida infection has developed, with the white itchy discharge that is usually fairly typical of it, there are several things that can be done.

To begin with, a visit to the surgery is worthwhile because your doctor can prescribe an antifungal cream or pessaries, containing drugs such as nystatin, isoconazole nitrate and clotrimazole, and can give tablets to help prevent reinfection. Incidentally, it is often wise for a woman's male partner to have a course of antifungal tablets. Even if he hasn't got any symptoms at all he may still be a carrier.

Home-grown treatment includes washing with a solution of one teaspoonful of vinegar in a pint of water, painting the affected area with aqueous gentian violet and eating plenty of plain yoghurt. Eating plain yoghurt sounds rather silly, but in fact yoghurt contains lactobacilli which compete with, and oust, the infection. Many women have reported a reduction in symptoms after dipping tampons in plain yoghurt and placing them inside their vaginas. Don't use sweetened strawberry rich yoghurts because they'll probably make things worse.

Finally, candida can be transmitted along with other infections such as gonorrhoea and trichomonas. If you suspect that you've acquired your candida as a sexually transmitted disease then do visit a specialist clinic for a check-up.

See also Hygiene (p. 40), Sexually transmitted diseases (p. 74) and Trichomonas (p. 81)

16

CERVICAL CAP

It looks a bit like a large thimble and fits over the cervix to prevent sperm passing out of the vagina and into the uterus. It is a simple but remarkably effective form of barrier contraception. If put into position before intercourse starts and left there for about six hours afterwards the cervical cap has a failure rate of about two in every hundred woman years. That means that if one hundred women use the cap for a year and have intercourse regularly then two of them will get pregnant. Alternatively, if one woman uses the cap for a hundred years then she has a two per cent chance of getting pregnant! That's a pretty low failure rate which compares well with some forms of contraceptive pill and intra-uterine device. The main advantage with the cervical cap is that it has no side effects. Its other advantage, and the one which makes it preferable to the condom or sheath, is that it doesn't interfere with either partner's pleasure. In addition to mechanically obstructing the passage of sperm into the uterus, by the way, the cervical cap (or Dutch cap as it is sometimes known) also works by preventing cervical secretions reaching the vagina. These cervical secretions are important because they help to neutralise the pH of the vagina and therefore help the sperm to survive in an otherwise hostile environment. (Nature really is very clever. The vagina needs to be acidic in order to make sure that infective organisms cannot survive. But that acidity is temporarily neutralised during intercourse so that conception can take place.)

Women who use cervical caps don't usually take long to learn how to pop them into position and some have found that they have one unique advantage over other forms of contraception. If put into position during an inconvenient period the flow of blood can be temporarily halted. When the cap is subsequently removed the blood is then released.

The latest development in cervical caps can't be used that way, however. An American doctor has developed a cervical cap which needs to be custom-made to fit on to a woman's cervix. It is fitted with a small one-way valve which allows menstrual fluid to flow out but which doesn't allow sperm to get in. Cervical mucus is presumably too sticky to get through the valve in useful quantities. The advantage of this type of cap is that it can be left in position for up to a year at a time.

Cervical caps have been rather ignored in the past. I think they could prove to have a big future as safe, effective and trouble-free forms of contraception.

See also Contraception (p. 22)

CERVICAL EROSION

The symptoms are usually no more than a watery discharge and some bleeding after intercourse. When the cervix is examined with the aid of a speculum it will be seen to be rather red. It is a problem that is common among young women, particularly those taking the contraceptive pill, and it is one that will often go away by itself without any treatment. When the symptoms don't resolve they can usually be cured with cautery, cryosurgery or diathermy. The cervical erosion is nothing to do with cancer of the cervix and it is not anything to worry about.

See also Cervix (p. 19)

CERVICAL SMEAR

By examining cells taken from the surface of the cervix it is sometimes possible to tell when ordinary, healthy cells are changing into cancer cells. Called a smear because it involves 'smearing' a collection of cells across a glass slide, this test is a now widely used screening procedure.

When the sample cells are examined under a microscope there are several possibilities. Sometimes it is clear that there is a real problem there and medical intervention is urgently required. Usually, of course, there is absolutely no problem at all. And occasionally there are minor abnormalities which might or might not turn out to produce a problem in the future. In this latter case it is safe to leave things alone and to re-examine another sample in six to twelve months' time. By then the cells will usually indicate that some action should be taken or that everything has returned to normal.

Although this particular screening test has undoubtedly picked up many early cancers and has saved a number of lives there is still some confusion about just when the test should be done. One widely held feeling is that all women should have a cervical smear done once every five years after their first sexual experience.

See also Cancer (p. 11)

CERVIX

The mouth of the uterus which projects into the innermost end of the vagina and which can be felt with the fingertips. The opening in the cervix (through which sperm must swim before an egg can be fertilised) is normally quite narrow but during childbirth the opening dilates to allow the baby to pass through.

See also Anatomy (p. 6), Cervical cap (p. 17), Cervical erosion (p. 18), Cervical smear (p. 18), Uterus (p. 82)

CHLAMYDIA

Chlamydia trachomatis is a common parasite. Its a bug that causes trachoma – a devastating eye disease – but which is also responsible for about fifty per cent of all cases of non-specific urethritis. Chlamydia is said to be the commonest cause of a sexually transmitted disease.

The initial symptoms of infection with chlamydia include abdominal pain and a vaginal discharge. Later salpingitis is a real risk. One of the reasons why the infection is so common is that women often have no symptoms at all in the early stages.

Chlamydia infection can be treated with antibiotics such as tetracycline, co-trimoxazole or erythromycin.

See also Sexually transmitted diseases (p. 74)

CIRCUMCISION

Circumcision, an operation which involves the surgical removal of the foreskin, is usually thought of as an operation performed solely on males. It isn't. Female circumcision is now a very well established ritual in many parts of the world and one which is done far too often.

Back in the nineteenth century female circumcision was performed in the Western world for all sorts of reasons. It was done for nervous disorders and all types of sexual problems, it was done for hysteria, epilepsy, masturbation, alleged nymphomania and such vague problems as 'moist palms'. The operation was done on seamstresses who operated treadle sewing machines and who found the sexual stimulation produced by their thighs rubbing together too much to bear. And it was done when doctors couldn't think of what else to do.

To-day clitoridectomy (and female circumcision) usually involves the removal of whole organs and not just the trimming of loose skin) is usually done for religious, social or sexual reasons. Despite the fact that there is no logical medical reasons for circumcision the operation is performed on millions of healthy women every year.

The operation described as 'female circumcision' may involve the removal of one or more of these: the clitoris, the clitoral prepuce, the labia minora, and the labia majora. The consequences include infection, bleeding, infertility, and a whole host of sexual problems.

CLITORIS

The most sensitive part of a woman's body and the female equivalent of the penis. Situated at the point where the two labia minora meet above the vaginal opening the clitoris is composed of erectile tissue and it enlarges when touched or stimulated in any way. It is stimulation of the clitoris that produces an orgasm.

See also Anatomy (p. 6), G spot (p. 36), Orgasm (p. 54)

COLPOSCOPY

In order to examine the cervix properly doctors sometimes use a colposcope – an instrument which is a low power microscope, magnifying five to ten times, but which can be used together with a vaginal speculum. It can be used without an anaesthetic.

CONDOMS

Also known as 'sheaths' (and various other things) condoms have been the butt of many jokes over the years. Using them has been compared to 'paddling with Wellington boots on' or 'playing the piano with gloves on' and it has frequently been suggested that having sex with a layer of rubber separating the penis from the vagina is worse than no sex at all.

Despite all this, however, condoms are still widely used. Some 40 million couples use them regularly and in Japan and China condoms are very much leading forms of contraception. Today, companies make condoms in many different shapes and colours and you can buy products that are straight or contoured, smooth or ribbed, transparent or coloured and thin or very thin. You can buy them with or without teats at the end to hold the sperm. And you can buy them with or without a lubricant added. You can even buy hypo-allergenic sheaths should you or your partner be unduly sensitive. Condoms stretch so easily (at least 600 per cent – you can even blow them up like balloons) that only one size is made, and that will fit organs of all descriptions. They're also pretty tough although they can, of course, be torn by teeth or finger nails.

Despite the fact that some people find them distasteful, condoms do have a number of advantages. They're convenient, they don't produce any side effects, they're useful for emergency, short-term use, they help delay orgasms when the male partner suffers from premature ejaculation, they're inexpensive, they can be used by either partner (he can carry one in his wallet or she can carry one in her handbag) and they're easy to get hold of without a prescription.

The other main advantage of a condom is that it also provides some protection against infection. The sheath not only reduces the risk of venereal disease being contracted but it also reduces the risk of pelvic inflammatory disease developing later. There is even evidence that if condoms are used regularly they reduce a woman's chances of developing cancer of the cervix.

If put on to the penis as soon as it becomes erect and removed after ejaculation and before the penis becomes limp again condoms are very efficient and effective contraceptives. Artificial lubricants shouldn't be used with condoms, by the way, because they may weaken the material.

Used properly the pregnancy risks associated with condom use are slight. If a hundred women rely on condoms for a year then no more than one or two should get pregnant. That's a failure rate comparable with the mini pill, the intra-uterine contraceptive device and other forms of barrier protection. Failures, when they occur, are usually due to over-eagerness, carelessness or tears produced by sharp finger nails or teeth!

See also Contraception (p. 22)

CONTRACEPTION

The chances of a woman getting pregnant after a single, isolated instance of intercourse seem to be approximately one in five. For those couples who want to limit their family, and those who don't want a family at all, some form of contraception is obviously needed if the odds are to be improved.

There are a number of different forms of contraception available and before making a choice consumers should look at the acceptability, effectiveness and side effects of the methods which can be used. Aesthetic qualities must be balanced against failure rates and it has to be remembered that a method one or both partners find unpleasant to use will probably not be used on every occasion and therefore its effectiveness will be reduced.

Whatever form of contraception is selected it must be remembered that if the method isn't used 'as directed' then the failure rate will probably increase.

When used properly the most efficient contraceptive is probably the combined pill (which contains both oestrogen and progestogen). This pill has a failure rate of less than one in a hundred woman years. In other words if a hundred women take the pill for a year and have sex fairly regularly, the chances are against more than one of them getting pregnant. The mini pill (progestogen-only pill), the intra-uterine contraceptive device, the condom, the cap and the diaphragm come next with a pregnancy rate of two in every hundred women years while such alternatives as the rhythm method, the withdrawal method and spermicides come last with an unacceptably high pregnancy rate approaching twenty per cent.

The main forms of contraception discussed elsewhere in this book are:

In addition researchers are currently experimenting with dozens of other new techniques. A male pill is still being talked about, a nasal spray contraceptive is an apparently genuine alternative and a sponge soaked with a spermicide is an unlikely but seemingly effective possibility.

CUNNILINGUS

Cunnilingus is oral sex concentrating on, in or around the vaginal area. It is an extremely common and safe sexual practice but there are one or two possible problems worth watching out for. So, for example, if medicated creams or pessaries have been used then the person performing cunnilingus may absorb the active ingredients quite unintentionally.

Blowing into the vagina can cause problems by pushing air into the peritoneal cavity. Blowing into the vagina of a pregnant woman is particularly likely to be dangerous since it can put air emboli into the large blood vessels – and that can kill.

Finally, it is worth remembering that although saliva is spermicidal cunnilingus can (if it follows fellatio and kissing in the right order) result in a conception.

CYST

A cyst is an enlargement or swelling that is usually filled with fluid. Ovaries commonly develop cysts which can vary from the size of a grape to the size of a melon. Most cysts are harmless but they can occasionally produce problems. So, for example, ovarian cysts can twist, rupture or bleed.

CYSTITIS

Cystitis – literally an inflammation of the bladder – is extremely common. Every year something like one in every five women suffer from it. Although men can, and do, suffer from cystitis women are particularly susceptible because they have very short urethras. The female urethral opening is close to the vagina and to the anus. It is, therefore, relatively easy for the urethra to be damaged during intercourse or to be infected by bugs living on one or both of the other passages.

Pain on passing urine, and having to pass small amounts of urine quite frequently are the two symptoms most commonly associated with the problem. Other common signs include the passing of cloudy or bloodstained urine.

Any cystitis sufferer should read the following pieces of advice:

1 Whenever you need to pass urine try and do so as soon as you can. If you delay too long then you may exacerbate an existing problem.

2 Cystitis can be caused or made worse by concentrated fruit juices, acid-tasting fruits, sweet foods, spicy foods, tea, coffee, alcohol, etc.

3 There is often a strong link between cystitis and sex. There is even a variation on the single theme, known as 'Honeymoon cystitis'. To minimise the risk of problems both partners should wash themselves before sex and women should wash afterwards. A French bidet is all you need – internal washouts are not necessary. The area should then be dabbed dry. If the vagina is dry then a lubricant is a good idea too.

4 Anyone suffering from cystitis should drink huge amounts of fluid – preferably plain water. Three or four pints a day are needed to help wash out the bladder and urethra. Sufferers who are already visiting the lavatory several times an hour think this sounds crazy but in fact they won't have to pass urine any more often but they will pass a greater quantity. And that will help to wash out any bugs that are there.

5 The bugs that cause cystitis prefer acidic urine. You can make urine slightly alkaline by drinking a solution of one teaspoonful of bicarbonate of soda every three or four hours. Don't do this for more than a day or so because the bicarbonate of soda can eventually produce problems of its own. Potassium citrate liquid or tablets can also be used.

6 When wiping themselves women should always wipe from front to back – and never from back to front. After passing a motion the natural tendency is often to wipe from the anus towards the urethra. That simply spreads infection. Do it in the opposite direction.

7 Personal hygiene in the whole vulva area is important but all you ever need use is warm water and a soft towel. Deodorants and antiseptics cause more problems than they cure.

8 If the symptoms of cystitis persist for more than a day or two then a urine test is often a good idea. If any bugs can be identified

then a suitable antibiotic can be prescribed. On balance, however, most cystitis sufferers will probably get better without an antibiotic. Its worth remembering that after using an antibiotic many women develop a vaginal infection.

See also Honeymoon cystitis (p. 40), Midstream specimen (p. 53)

D & C

The female uterus has a lining which is many cells deep and every month, as the levels of circulating hormones vary, so the number of cells making up that lining increases and decreases. When a woman ovulates her uterus prepares a special cell lining just in case the egg gets fertilised. When the egg isn't fertilised then the lining is discarded – as a menstrual period. Since most women start to menstruate by the time they are fifteen years of age and carry on menstruating until they're about forty-five that means that the monthly building up and breaking down of cells will go on for thirty years. Even allowing for a pregnancy or two that means that an average sort of woman can expect to renew the lining to her uterus several hundred times.

It is perhaps not surprising, therefore, that the normal, regular menstrual pattern sometimes gets disturbed. Sometimes periods are too light. Sometimes they are too heavy. Occasionally they are too close together. On other occasions they are too far apart. There is sometimes too much accompanying pain. And so on and so on. The difficulty lies in the fact that when things do go wrong the clues and solutions often lie among the cells in the uterus. The only way to find out exactly what is going on – and why things are going wrong – is to take a specimen of the cells which line the womb.

And that's probably the commonest sort of reason for a D & C – a dilatation and curettage.

The D & C is a fairly simple and straightforward operation to perform. It usually takes about ten minutes under a general anaesthetic. After first measuring the length of the whole cavity with a specially marked rod (to make sure that he doesn't inadvertently push any of his instruments through the vagina and uterus and into the abdominal cavity) the gynaecologist will begin by enlarging the size of the cervix, the narrow opening that leads into the uterus. Under normal circumstances the cervix has such a narrow opening that to try and examine the cell lining of the uterus without enlarging it would be like trying to clean out the living room with the door shut and only the keyhole to work through.

The instruments used to enlarge the cervix are called dilators. They are usually made of steel, they are long, thin and round ended. The operating gynaecologist will usually begin with a very thin dilator and gradually work his way up to one large enough to dilate the cervix wide enough for him to work through it. It will usually take half a dozen dilators of gradually increasing sizes to get to that stage. Fortunately for gynaecologists the cervix, unlike a keyhole, is fairly easy to dilate. It is, after all, built to expand far enough to let a baby through!

Once the cervix has been dilated the surgeon will reach for a curette; an instrument that looks a bit like a long handled ice-cream spoon – the sort of thing they give you so that you can finish the last bit of your Knickerbocker Glory. By pushing the curette in through the dilated cervix the gynaecologist can then either take a sample from the womb lining or he can systematically clean out the whole of the lining. Given the name of the instrument that is used it is hardly surprising that this procedure is called curettage. It's all a bit like scraping the innards out of an avocado pear.

Once samples have been obtained from the lining these will usually be sent along to the laboratory where they can be examined under a microscope. The whole procedure won't have taken more than a few minutes, it won't involve more than one or possibly two days in hospital, and it shouldn't have any nasty after-effects.

A D & C has two main uses. First, by providing samples of the cells inside the womb it helps gynaecologists decide precisely why problems have developed. And second it sometimes seems to eradicate symptoms. I don't think anyone knows why it works so often. But it does. Perhaps the womb lining just builds up and needs a good clean out occasionally.

There are other reasons for doing a D & C too. It can be done if a woman is infertile (in which case it can help provide valuable information which might provide clues as to why she hasn't got pregnant) and it can be done when a woman who doesn't want to be pregnant is (in which case it ends the pregnancy).

See also Aspiration curettage (p. 8)

DIAPHRAGM

A contraceptive device made of soft rubber and usually fitted with a metal spring. The diaphragm fits inside the vagina and acts as a mechanical barrier stopping sperm reaching the womb.

See also Contraception (p. 22)

DISCHARGES

Some form of vaginal discharge is quite normal. The vagina produces its own lubricating fluids which keep the tissues moist and free of infection and which make intercourse more comfortable. The amount of discharge normally produced varies from woman to woman and will usually be at a maximum during puberty, during pregnancy or when a woman is taking the contraceptive pill. The amount of discharge produced normally is dependent upon the amount of circulating hormones and hormone production goes up at puberty and during pregnancy and is artificially raised when the pill is being taken.

A vaginal discharge usually only becomes a problem if it is offensive, itchy, irritating or so profuse that it necessitates either the wearing of a pad or the constant changing of clothes. When that happens the commonest explanation is that there is a local infection (such as candida or trichomonas or an infection of a cervical erosion) or that some foreign body (usually a forgotten tampon) has been left in the vagina and is producing an irritation. Venereal infections are also a possible explanation and sometimes these same symptoms can be produced by the use of deodorants or antiseptics which themselves produce a local dermatitis, inflammation, irritation and increase in discharge.

The treatment of the discharge will naturally depend on the cause. To find out exactly what is causing the problem an examination will usually be necessary and unless the cause is very clear and easily treatable a swab will usually have to be sent to the laboratory for testing. Only then will the precise cause of any infection be identifiable.

DOCTORS

Many women with what are often politely known as 'personal' problems or 'troubles down below' fail to get the best out of their doctors because they are too shy or embarrassed to seek help at the right time, ask the right questions, provide all the important bits and pieces of information or even answer straightforward questions.

Read and follow *this* advice and you'll be sure to get a good deal out of your doctor when you visit him with a 'personal matter'.

1 Don't delay. Whatever it is that is worrying you may go away. But it may not. So you might as well get it dealt with now. You might have to wait for a few days if you insist on seeing a specific doctor. If you think it could be urgent (and if you're worried about it then it's urgent) settle for an appointment with any doctor. And insist on being seen today or tomorrow. They'll fit you in. If the receptionist claims that they can't see you for a week ask to speak to the doctor on the telephone. If she says you can't then insist on a home visit. And if the doctor doesn't approve of your tactics then change to another practice.

2 Be prepared for an examination. You're probably going to need to be examined sooner or later. You wouldn't expect your doctor to deal with a problem affecting your hands without getting you to remove your gloves, would you? Dress in something fairly simple if you can. Stockings are easier than tights and zips are quicker for nervous, fumbling fingers than lots of fiddly buttons.

When it comes to the examination some doctors do it with a chaperone present. Others don't. If you feel strongly about it either way tell him. Apart from putting two fingers inside your vagina he'll probably want to take a look inside with the aid of a speculum. That way he'll be able to see as well as feel if there is anything wrong. It might be unpleasant or uncomfortable but it shouldn't hurt. If it does, then tell him.

Don't be surprised if he wants to put a finger into your rectum as well. He may want to put fingers into both openings at once. It helps to examine things from two different angles.

If he thinks there could be an infection he will probably take a swab. That just means taking a sample of any discharge on a king-sized cotton bud. If you haven't had a smear done recently he may do that too. It doesn't mean that he suspects anything. It's just routine.

3 Don't for heaven's sake chicken out. Don't be shy. Don't worry about shocking or embarrassing your doctor. You won't be able to. Mention your problem as soon as you get into the surgery. Don't chicken out and complain about a slight cough or a bunion at the last minute. GPs are well aware that many patients who complain of trivial ailments really want to talk about something else. But few doctors are likely to start asking you about your vagina unless you at least give a hint in that direction!

4 Make your mind up beforehand about what you want to tell him. If you think you're likely to forget things then write down your symptoms, signs and complaints on a piece of paper. And do take along details of your last few periods. He's bound to ask you about your periods and if you have to hunt through your diary you'll probably get all flustered and forget other things you wanted to say.

5 Don't be startled or offended at any questions he asks. If you have a discharge your doctor will want to know how long you've had it, what colour it is, whether or not it is bloodstained, whether it smells, whether there is any itching, whether the discharge is thick or watery, whether it has changed recently and whether you've had anything like it before. He'll want to know whether you take the contraceptive pill, whether you've had any pains or bleeding or other symptoms and what your periods are like. As a matter of routine he may want to know how often you have intercourse, whether it hurts, whether you could be pregnant and if you could have contracted a sexually transmitted disease. All those are perfectly routine questions.

6 Decide in advance what questions you want to ask your doctor. Write down the questions you would like to have answered if you think you're likely to forget any of them. And do ask about anything

you don't understand. Your family doctor is the one person you should be able to ask about anything. If you've been to the hospital and a gynaecologist has used a term or word you don't know then ask your family doctor. One of his jobs is to act as an interpreter.

7 Write down anything your doctor tells you to do. Doctors write down things patients tell them because they'll forget otherwise. And there is absolutely no reason why patients shouldn't write things down too. Take a notepad and pencil with you and jot down anything that sounds useful or important.

8 At the end of your consultation be sure you know exactly what you have got to do. Have you got to stop taking the contraceptive pill for a month? Have you got to avoid intercourse for a week? Have you got to ring the hospital for an appointment? Have you got to return to the surgery in a week? Make sure you know what you have got to do – and if you're not sure then ask.

9 Don't worry if your doctor tells you that he is going to send you to see a specialist. It doesn't mean that he thinks that there is anything wrong. It simply means that he isn't sure of the diagnosis. Or that he wants help with the treatment. If when you get a hospital appointment it is for a date weeks or months ahead then let your family doctor know – by shopping around among different hospitals and different specialists it's often possible to obtain an earlier appointment.

10 If at the end of your consultation you aren't happy about the way things have gone then ask for a second opinion. You're entitled to one. If your own doctor won't arrange a second opinion for you then just ring another doctor and make an appointment to see him. If, on the other hand, you're happy with what your doctor has done and said then do follow his advice and instructions!

See also Gynaecologists (p. 38), Obstetricians (p. 54)

DOUCHING

Douching, or washing out the vagina, is done for all sorts of reasons. It is done to stop infection developing. It's done to stop pregnancy. And it is done as a sort of semi-religious ritual to prevent disease, discharge and bad odour. It is done with plain water, with antiseptic solutions, with special commercial preparations and with solutions prepared according to recipes handed down from mother to daughter.

It is, however, unnecessary and ineffective.

It doesn't make any real difference to an infection that is likely to develop. And it certainly won't have much effect on a woman's chances of getting pregnant.

The vagina is, in fact, very well designed for looking after itself. A continuous supply of secretions make their way towards the entrance and help to conquer and deal with bugs of all kinds. Douching is simply likely to push infections further up the vagina and to oppose the body's own protective mechanisms.

As for douching to prevent pregnancy – well, it is difficult to be sure that a douching procedure wouldn't push sperm further up towards the cervix rather than wash them back out again.

See also Contraception (p. 22), Hygiene (p. 40)

DRUGS

The only creams, ointments, wipes, pessaries, suppositories, tablets or sprays that should be used in or around the vagina are ones prescribed by a doctor. Medicines sold over the counter (without a prescription) for vaginal problems of any kind are unlikely to help but may produce rashes, infections and allergy reactions.

Drugs taken orally for problems down below are only suitable for short-term use. Any problem which persists or recurs needs professional treatment. Over the counter preparations sold for period problems are unlikely to offer lasting relief and may produce side effects.

DYSMENORRHOEA

Painful periods.

See also Period problems (p. 59)

DYSPAREUNIA

Painful sexual intercourse.

See also Sexual problems (p. 72)

ECTOPIC PREGNANCY

Normally when a sperm meets and fertilises an egg the resulting embryo develops in the womb. Occasionally, however, things go wrong and the developing foetus settles not in the womb but in one of the Fallopian tubes. That's an ectopic pregnancy and it is likely to cause abdominal pains, bleeding, nausea and faintness.

An ectopic pregnancy is a possibility that must be considered whenever a pregnant woman develops unexpected abdominal pain.

ENDOMETRIOSIS

Each month the cells which make up the lining of the womb (the endometrium) build up under hormonal control. Then, if no egg is fertilised, the lining breaks down and the discharge of the cells from the womb produces the monthly bleeding that characterises a woman's reproductive years.

Problems can occur if the endometrial tissue is present outside the womb. If, for example, endometrial tissue is attached to the outer sides of the womb itself, is wrapped around one or both ovaries or is fixed in the pelvis then that tissue will respond to the monthly build-up of hormones in exactly the same way as the endometrial tissue inside the womb.

The cells will get thicker and thicker and finally, after expanding to their collective limit, they will break down and bleed.

Inside the womb the bleeding isn't a problem. The blood simply passes out through the cervix and the vagina and is discharged from the body. When the endometrial tissue is on the other side of the womb wall, however, problems arise. The blood can't escape as a period bleed can. It builds up and forms cysts. And there is often a considerable amount of pain. Indeed pain is probably the most important and commonest single symptom of endometriosis. There is pain at period time, pain during intercourse and general pain for no very apparent reason at all.

Precisely why endometrial tissue develops in these wayward places is something of a mystery but we do know that all the symptoms associated with endometriosis are very much under hormonal control. Women who have reached the menopause don't have any more problems. Nor do women who for some reason don't have normal monthly bleeding.

More important perhaps it is also known that pregnancy seems to be an effective treatment for endometriosis. The disorder rarely affects women who have had children and when a sufferer gets pregnant the problem usually disappears. Since getting pregnant is a rather extreme form of treatment it is possible to imitate the hormonal changes by using a hormone pill – and to end the symptoms of endometriosis with equal efficiency.

Occasionally, hormone treatment (whether through a natural pregnancy or some form of hormone pill) doesn't work and the endometriosis persists. When that happens the sufferer may need an operation to remove some of the extraneous tissue.

Endometriosis isn't always easy to diagnose but it is a fairly common problem. It should always be thought of as a possible diagnosis whenever any woman (and particularly a woman who hasn't ever been pregnant) develops strange pains in or around the pelvis or lower abdomen, or develops pains which are worse either at period time or during sexual intercourse.

See also Period problems (p. 59), Uterus (p. 82)

EPISIOTOMY

Although the tissues around the outside of the vagina can stretch a great deal they cannot always stretch enough to allow a baby to pass through. When the skin tissues are over-stretched there is a risk that a tear will result.

To avoid an untidy and possibly difficult-to-heal skin rip an obstetrician will sometimes make a quite deliberate cut at the bottom end of the vagina. This then enlarges the gap available for the baby to pass through and because the cut will have neat, straight edges it will be easy to sew up again.

This cut is called an episiotomy.

FALLOPIAN TUBES

Slender, fairly narrow tubes which project from either side of the uterus and which end somewhere near the two ovaries. Eggs from the ovaries pass along the two Fallopian tubes and into the uterus.

Infection and inflammation can damage the tubes and make a woman infertile by preventing eggs from reaching the womb.

See also Anatomy (p. 6), Ovaries (p. 55), Sterilisation (p. 75) and Uterus (p. 82)

FIBROIDS

The normal, healthy uterus is made up of a huge number of powerful muscle fibres. Although no one really knows why they do it these fibres can occasionally grow too much, forming muscle tumours known as myomata, or fibroids.

Benign, and more of a nuisance than a real threat or danger, these fibroids can sometimes grow to the size of a grapefruit. Usually they keep to something much more modest – say the size of a plum or small orange. If they're big enough they can be felt from the outside and if they're really big they can make a woman look pregnant.

Apart from their size fibroids fall into one or two main categories: the ones which grow into the lining of the womb, and which can therefore affect a woman's periods, and the ones which remain within the wall of the uterus. Fibroids which grow into the womb lining, which may produce quite heavy bleeding even if they're fairly small, are known as sub-mucous or interstitial fibroids.

Fibroids which remain within the womb wall are known as sub-serous. They sometimes fail to produce any symptoms at all.

All in all, about one in every five women end up growing fibroids at some time of life or another. The problem is commoner in women who haven't had children, or who have had children late in life.

Fibroids can be dealt with in one or two ways. They can either be removed surgically (sometimes tricky and not always successful since more fibroids can always develop) or they can be removed together with the whole womb.

A myomectomy (or the specific removal of the fibroid) is obviously the most suitable operation in a young woman and is a 'must' in a woman who wants to have future pregnancies. A hysterectomy may be suitable for the woman who is absolutely certain that she isn't going to want any more children.

See also Hysterectomy (p. 41), Uterus (p. 82)

FOREIGN OBJECTS IN THE VAGINA

Foreign objects in the vagina can cause a profuse, purulent, blood-stained discharge. Objects left in the vagina vary a great deal but include tampons, thermometers, coins, toys and all sorts of other bits and pieces. Doctors have reported finding bottles, beer glasses, compasses, bobbins, hairpins, goblets, needles, goldfish, gear lever knobs and a front collar stud. Pessaries used to hold weakened tissues in place are often left far too long and the record seems to be held by a woman who had a ring pessary in her vagina for a total of fifty-five years.

See also Hygiene (p. 40)

G SPOT

The G stands for Grafenberg, a German gynaecologist. Back in the 1940s, when he was researching different methods of birth control, Ernst Grafenberg, assiduous and observant, discovered what he described as a bean-shaped patch of erectile tissue in the front wall of the vagina. It was, according to his instructions, directly behind the pubic bone.

Grafenberg described this bean-shaped patch as a sort of second clitoris. He claimed that when stimulated by pressure on this spot women had what he described as a vaginal orgasm.

More recently three American authors, Ladas, Whipple and Perry have claimed that the G spot is a sort of female prostate gland and it has even been argued that the spot, patch or gland secretes a special fluid during orgasm, a claim which has given rise to the suggestion that women may really ejaculate when they reach a climax.

There is still some confusion about whether or not the G spot really exists, how it works and precisely what its function is. Gynaecologists who still haven't identified the spot claim that to look for it would be distinctly unethical and professionally hazardous since if they found it their patients might get the wrong idea. Pathologists, who have claimed that they haven't been able to find the bean-shaped patch when dissecting cadavers have been told that the G spot atrophies in older women.

Perhaps, when it comes down to it, it's the looking for the G spot that matters. Rather than the finding.

See also Anatomy (p. 6), Clitoris (p. 20), Orgasm (p. 54), Sexual problems (p. 72)

GONORRHOEA

Sixty per cent of the women who contract this sexually transmitted disease have no symptoms at all. The rest usually notice fairly vague and non-specific symptoms such as a vaginal discharge, burning on passing urine and a need to pass urine frequently. A few sufferers have pain in the pelvic region. The incubation period for the disease is between two and ten days and so when symptoms are going to develop it's usually within that sort of time range.

Diagnosing gonorrhoea is important for several reasons; it can produce pelvic inflammatory disease in sufferers and if they get pregnant and give birth while infected it can produce a very nasty form of eye inflammation in babies. Gonorrhoea is, of course, a very infectious disease and can easily be spread to sexual partners.

Once the diagnosis has been made the treatment will usually consist of penicillin.

See also Sexually transmitted diseases (p. 74)

GYNAECOLOGIST

A doctor who specialises in the treatment of women's problems.

See also Doctor (p. 29), Obstetrician (p. 54)

HAEMATURIA

Haematuria means blood in the urine and it can be caused by infection (such as cystitis) and by kidney stones. Apparent haematuria is sometimes produced when urine gets mixed with menstrual blood; or after the eating of substances like beetroot (which dye the urine red).

Although there is often no identifiable cause for haematuria it is a symptom which should always be investigated.

HERPES

In contrast to cold sores which are caused by the Herpes Simplex type I virus, genital herpes, a sexually transmitted disease, is caused by Herpes Simplex type II virus.

The initial symptoms of this disease which has, in recent years, affected hundreds of thousands and worried millions more, include such vague problems as headache, backache, fever and enlarged lymph nodes. Vaginal soreness and irritation are fairly common too, but the most specific complaint is usually the development of red blistery spots on and around the vulva. These will eventually turn into ulcers and will usually become painful and cause pain when urine is passed.

The symptoms of genital herpes can begin anything between a day or two and a week after the infection has been contracted but they usually come and go after that. Typically the first attack of ulceration lasts between one and six weeks, then disappearing only to reappear at intervals of approximately one month for years afterwards. The open sores are the greatest source of infection but sufferers do remain infectious during *and* between acute attacks. Incidentally there is also evidence that the herpes virus can exist for several hours on lavatory seats, and so this is one sexually transmitted disease which can be picked up without having intercourse.

The pain, discomfort and embarrassment caused by herpes are bad enough but there is now also evidence linking the herpes infection to cancer of the cervix. In addition there is a risk that any babies born to infected mothers will suffer and perhaps die as a result.

Since herpes is a fairly straightforward venereal disease it is obviously best avoided simply by avoiding intercourse with individuals who may be infected. It is, however, also true that condoms and spermicidal creams do seem to offer some protection. It is also worth remembering that the infection can only be passed on by direct contact.

Once the herpes infection has been caught there are several remedies which can be tried. The anti-viral agent acycloguanosine is sometimes said to help and four per cent or eight per cent lithium chloride in ointment base is also claimed to have useful properties for relieving the symptoms produced by acute attacks. Salt baths are also sometimes recommended. Wearing loose clothes and resting during the most exhaustive periods of the infection are additional pieces of advice worth following.

The most exciting breakthrough in the prevention and treatment of herpes genitalis involves a new vaccine which has been developed. This has been tried on sufferers and on their uninfected partners and it seems that two jabs may help prevent the disease developing while three may cure the disease once it has taken hold. The vaccine is not yet widely available but progress in this area is being made rapidly.

See also Sexually transmitted disease (p. 74)

HONEYMOON CYSTITIS

'Honeymoon cystitis' is the rather delicate phrase used to describe cystitis associated with sexual intercourse. It certainly isn't confined to brides. Sex causes bladder problems for two reasons: either because intercourse has been rather too energetic and the female urethra has been subjected to a physical battering, or because infection has been passed on.

The problem can be avoided, or at least minimised, by experimenting with different positions (in an attempt to find ones which do not result in the urethra being traumatised) and by taking care with personal hygiene. Both partners should wash themselves before sex and women should empty their bladders after sex to make sure that any bacteria around the urethra are washed away.

Finally, the problem can sometimes also be minimised if a pillow is placed beneath the female partner's buttocks when the missionary position is being used.

See also Cystitis (p. 24)

HYGIENE

Bad odours and vaginal discharges are sometimes caused by sweating, retained tampons, old blood, infections, skin fold infestations, old semen and smegma and other similar problems.

Because of a desperate (if natural) urge to avoid developing smells and discharges many women use special talcum powders, deodorant sprays, medicated wipes and other commercial products. Not only are these products a waste of money but they are also a potential hazard. Antiseptics and deodorants used around the vulval area cause soreness and irritation, allergies and rashes. Ironically they can even result in infections developing.

It is much wiser to keep the vulval area clean simply by following simple rules of personal hygiene. The area should be washed daily in a bath or bidet, using a plain soap and plenty of warm water. Perfumed soaps should be avoided since they can cause problems too. Stockings, loose fitting cotton panties or paper panties are better than tights, nylon panties or close fitting, figure hugging bikini panties. If problems persistently develop then panties shouldn't be worn at all. (Oddly enough this suggestion sometimes seems to startle women who would happily go without a bra but who think going without panties vaguely indecent.) Shaving away some of the pubic hair will help make it easier to keep the genital area clean and fresh.

HYMEN

A thin membrane which covers the external opening of the vagina in virgins. There is usually a small hole in the hymen through which menstrual blood can escape. If there is no such opening then blood will build up inside and produce a painful swelling.

The hymen is usually ruptured during intercourse but it may also be ruptured by using tampons, by bicycle riding or by horse riding.

See also Anatomy (p. 6)

HYSTERECTOMY

In most parts of the so-called developed world between one in two and one in five of all women will eventually have their wombs removed. This makes hysterectomy one of the commonest of all operations.

The operation is performed for several reasons. It is done for women who have heavy or irregular periods which cannot be controlled in any other way, it is done for women who have inexplicable pelvic pain, who have fibroids, who have a prolapse, who have bleeding between their periods or who have bleeding after the menopause. Relatively rarely cancer is the reason for hysterectomy.

The womb can be removed in one of two main ways. First, it can be removed by making an incision in the abdomen. Sometimes the cut is made vertically, running down from the umbilicus. More commonly it is made horizontally, in such a way that it will be hidden underneath the bottom half of a bikini. The bikini scar, as it is called, is not just done for cosmetic reasons – because it doesn't involve cutting through muscle layers it usually heals more easily.

Second, the womb can be removed from a vaginal approach. This technique, usually preferred when there is a bladder weakness to be repaired or a prolapse to be mended, doesn't leave a visible scar at all.

Both types of operation will usually necessitate a hospital stay of eight to ten days. After returning home the patient will usually need to rest for a week before slowly beginning to get back to a normal life. Four to six weeks are usually needed off work and most surgeons recommend that their patients avoid sexual inter-course for about six weeks – to give the area time to heal.

There are all sorts of myths and misconceptions about the hysterectomy operation. Many women, for example, fear that they will lose their femininity after such a procedure. That just isn't true at all. The womb doesn't produce any hormones and it is only if the ovaries are removed in addition to the uterus that there is any likelihood of obvious physical changes occurring. After a normal, straightforward hysterectomy the only thing a woman is really likely to notice is that she doesn't have any more periods. Without a womb there can't be any bleeding at all. Nor can a woman get pregnant.

Indeed surveys which have been done have shown that most women who have had their wombs taken out have felt better afterwards! One study showed that ninety-four per cent of women had sex lives which were just as good or even better after they had their wombs removed while ninety-seven per cent claimed that their health was better after a hysterectomy than it had been before. Three-quarters of all women who have had a hysterectomy are back to normal life three months after surgery.

One problem women do notice after a hysterectomy is that their vaginas are a little drier than usual. This happens because some secretions normally come down from the womb and cervix area. A little artificial lubrication with a cream or jelly is usually all that is needed although it is obviously wise for the male partner to be cautious, careful and gentle to begin with. If the womb has been removed through the vagina the entrance may be a little narrower than before too. Most women don't find this much of a problem!

Hysterectomy is a disaster when it is done on a woman who afterwards feels that she would have liked more children. There isn't much that can be done then and the regrets are likely to lead to heartache and even serious depression. For this reason it is important that every woman who is about to have a hysterectomy should think carefully about the consequences. If she thinks she might want more children at any future date then she should say so. Then, if there is any possible alternative to a total womb removal, it should be taken.

See also Sterilisation (p. 75), Uterus (p. 82)

INCONTINENCE OF URINE

Incontinence is an uncomfortable and extremely embarrassing problem that can have devastating effects. It is something that affects 10 per cent of all premenopausal women and 25 per cent of all postmenopausal women. It is therefore a major problem.

There are a number of possible causes. Sometimes a fistula or a congenital abnormality may result in a leakage of urine. Occasionally, if the bladder is not emptying properly, it will fill and then overflow to produce a steady, persistent dribble of urine. Not infrequently there is some instability in the muscles which causes incontinence and a need to pass urine at night. There is sometimes no real physical problem to be found at all. Drugs can sometimes be used to help patients with problems in these various categories and one particular product, emepronium bromide, is used widely to help individuals with mysterious bladder problems.

Probably the most important cause of urinary incontinence among women, however, is stress incontinence.

Normally urine is kept in the bladder by a valve or sphincter. When the bladder is full a message is relayed to the brain and, at a convenient moment, the sphincter is opened and urine released.

Sometimes, however, the urethral sphincter is too weak to hold urine in the bladder. Increases in the pressure inside the abdomen, and therefore increases in pressure inside the bladder, result in urine being forced past the sphincter and out through the urethral opening. Since the increase in pressure can be produced by such normal activities as laughing, crying, coughing or running it is easy to see just how embarrassing this particular problem can be.

The sphincter can become weakened in a number of ways. Having babies, for example, puts a tremendous strain on the muscles in that area and may eventually weaken them. Stress incontinence is often accompanied by a prolapse since both are due to muscle weakness in many women. Sometimes stress incontinence develops at the menopause as hormonal changes affect the body.

Occasionally the problem can be dealt with by deliberately strengthening the muscles around the sphincter with special exercises. (These are described on p. 57.) Often, however, it is necessary for a surgeon to operate and repair the weakness. In view of the social and mental traumas caused by stress incontinence, this is an operation usually well worth having.

See also Pelvic floor exercises (p. 57), Prolapse (p. 67)

INFERTILITY

Infertility is a problem that affects something like one couple in ten. Traditionally it's the female half of the partnership that is usually blamed when children aren't forthcoming but in practice the fault lies with the man just as often as it lies with the woman.

There are said to be approximately forty possible causes of infertility although you could probably find more if you looked hard enough. Among women the common problems are a failure of ovulation and a blockage of the Fallopian tubes (often caused by some previous infection) while among men the problems include a failure to produce spermatazoa in sufficient numbers, and a failure to produce spermatazoa of good enough quality. Those disorders can themselves be traced back to other problems in many cases. So, for example, when a woman fails to ovulate the cause may be a specific disorder such as endometriosis or a general complaint such as a considerable or sudden weight loss. When a man doesn't produce enough sperm or produces sperm of inferior quality the basic cause may be an old infection or even an accident. Mumps is a common enough cause of male sterility.

General illnesses such as diabetes mellitus and thyroid disorders can also cause infertility, past episodes of venereal disease can be responsible and occasionally one partner may develop anti-sperm antibodies.

It is also important to remember that infertility may be a result not of some internal failure but of a simple, straightforward failure to give spermatazoa a decent chance to meet an egg! So, for example, a man who is impotent or who prematurely ejaculates is unlikely to impregnate a woman. There are times too when a basic misunderstanding of human anatomy results in apparent infertility. I remember once seeing a couple who complained that they couldn't have any children but who turned out to have been trying to 'make a baby' by leaving sperm deposited in the woman's umbilicus. Another time I saw a couple who complained of child-lessness but who turned out to have mistakenly used the woman's urethra as a sperm depository. Technically she was still a virgin, with her hymen still intact, and all she had to show for several years of trying was a severe case of urinary incontinence. Finally, it is worth remembering that frequency of intercourse is also of some significance. The couple who make love once every three months are unlikely to have children as quickly as the couple who make love once every three days.

Generally speaking, unless a woman is over thirty years of age it isn't usually necessary to start investigating infertility until a couple have been having unprotected intercourse (i.e. not using any form of contraception) for two years.

And well before that time is reached there is quite a lot that a couple can do to enhance their chances of having a child.

Having sex as close as possible to the moment of ovulation is as good a starting point as any. Most women ovulate fourteen days before the end of their menstrual cycle so sex at that time is far more likely to result in a pregnancy than sex immediately before or immediately after a period. Sex during a period is particularly unlikely to result in conception since not only is there unlikely to be an egg around but also the womb lining isn't in any fit state to receive a fertilised egg. Incidentally any woman who menstruates regularly is unlikely not to be ovulating. The moment of ovulation can also be timed by keeping a record of the woman's body temperature. A slight fall and rise usually denotes ovulation.

To ensure that his sperm are kept in tiptop condition a man

should wear baggy shorts, avoid tight jeans, keep out of hot baths and hot saunas and sit with his legs apart whenever possible! Sperm are very susceptible to heat (that's why the testicles are suspended outside the body) and all these tips are designed to help keep the sperm as cool as possible.

After intercourse a woman who wants to get pregnant should stay in bed for half an hour, should draw her knees up and should perhaps even put a pillow under her bottom. These actions are designed to improve the chances of sperm getting into and through the cervix. The more sperm getting through into the womb the greater the chance of a pregnancy.

When, after two years of trying, there is still no hint of a pregnancy developing it is time to start investigating both partners. It is, of course, important for both partners to be tested since difficulties as commonly involve the man as the woman.

The course of action recommended will then, of course, depend on the nature of the problem. If a woman has two blocked Fallopian tubes then an operation may be possible to open them again. Fallopian tube transplantation is sometimes done. If a woman isn't ovulating then drugs such as clomiphene citrate can be used to stimulate ovulation. If a man isn't producing sperm in sufficient quantities then it may be possible to collect together the contents of several ejaculates and to artificially inseminate the woman when she ovulates. Sometimes, when the husband isn't producing sperm in sufficient quantities or is producing faulty sperm, an anonymous donor's sperm can be used instead. Finally infertility can sometimes be overcome by fertilising an egg outside a woman's body and then placing the growing embryo inside the womb – the 'test-tube baby' technique.

See also Artificial insemination (p. 8), Test-tube babies (p. 80)

INJECTABLE CONTRACEPTIVE

Hormonal contraceptive pills are very effective but they do have to be taken daily. Forget one pill and a pregnancy can result. There is, however, an alternative form of hormonal contraception which is available for those who find it difficult to remember to take a pill every day. The long lasting injection is called Depo-Provera and it slowly releases progestogen into the blood. This prevents the release of an egg and it alters the womb lining too.

Although it has been used for over fifteen years, has been used and approved by the World Health Organisation, has been given to women in all parts of the world and seems on the available evidence to be both safe and effective, the long lasting injectable contraceptive has aroused a good deal of opposition. Many of those opposing its use have done so not because of any specific medical problems associated with it but because of a fear that an injectable contraceptive might be given to women who were not aware of what was happening to them. They also make the point that once an injection has been given it may be difficult to reverse the effects until the normal life span of the injection has been reached.

On balance, the injectable contraceptive is probably best kept for those women who specifically ask for it because they recognise that they may have difficulty in remembering to take ordinary contraceptive pills.

See also Contraception (p. 22)

INTRA-UTERINE CONTRACEPTIVE DEVICE (IUCD)

It consists of a small piece of curved metal or plastic and it may come in any one of a number of different shapes and sizes. When put into the womb it prevents a woman getting pregnant, though just how it works is still something of a mystery.

The IUCD is a pretty effective contraceptive (figures suggest that about two out of every hundred women who use this method for a year will get pregnant) but it has had a pretty bad press in recent years. It can cause heavy bleeding, cramp-like pains and a discharge. Occasionally an IUCD may work its way through the wall of the womb and into the abdomen. It can sometimes produce severe pelvic infection. Sometimes it can come out of the womb. And, of course, there are those horror stories of babies being born triumphantly holding their mothers IUCDs in their tiny fists.

Those are the bad points.

It must also be pointed out, however, that many women have found IUCDs to be safe, comfortable and convenient. Once in place they don't need to be removed (although most doctors like them to be changed once every two years or so), they won't usually be dislodged by menstrual bleeding, tampons or sex, and they don't produce any general side effects.

IUCDs don't have to be remembered and they don't interfere with sexual satisfaction in any way. It's fairly easy to check that an IUCD is still in place by feeling for the thread that should poke out through the neck of the womb.

See also Contraception (p. 22)

ITCHING

There are many possible causes of itching in and around the vaginal area. Infections such as candida commonly cause itching as do allergy reactions to soap powder, new clothes, deodorant sprays, special creams and ointments and even the rubber of a contraceptive sheath. Generalised skin disorders, urinary incontinence, sexually transmitted diseases such as herpes and problems such as diabetes mellitus can also produce itching. In the very young and the fairly elderly, vaginal secretions are often inadequate and soreness is then a problem.

Since itching causes scratching and scratching causes bleeding there is also the problem that additional infections may develop. These may then, in turn, produce itching of their own. A real vicious circle!

To deal with this symptom effectively the basic cause must be dealt with first. While the primary problem is being dealt with, however, it is usually possible to get relief by using antihistamine tablets. These often cause drowsiness but they do relieve itching.

See also Discharges (p. 28), Hygiene (p. 40), Sexually transmitted disease (p. 74)

LABIA

The thin lips on both sides of the vaginal opening are known as the labia minora. The thicker, fat-filled lips outside the labia minora are known as the labia majora.

See also Anatomy (p. 6)

LAPAROTOMY

Making a cut in the abdominal wall and looking inside – done either to make a diagnosis or in order to provide treatment of some kind.

LAPAROSCOPY

A small incision is made in the abdominal wall so that the surgeon can look inside with a special telescope. It's a procedure done under a general anaesthetic but it can often be done on patients staying in hospital only for a day.

As a diagnostic procedure laparoscopy is done for unexplained pain and to investigate infertility. Sterilisation and the diathermy treatment of mild endometriosis can also be done through a laparoscopy incision.

LEUKOPLAKIA

White area of skin on and around the vulva which becomes thick, coarse and itchy. It splits and cracks and scratching may lead to infection.

LUMPS AND BUMPS

Lumps and bumps around the vagina may be caused by enlarged lymph nodes, boils or small cysts. Any lump that cannot easily be identified as entirely harmless should be examined by a doctor.

MASTURBATION

It doesn't cause blindness (or even short-sightedness), hairy palms, enlarged labia, madness or venereal diseases. It isn't a sign of immaturity and the only real problems associated with it are the feelings of guilt produced by the attitudes of others who are worried about their masturbatory habits. Learning how to masturbate successfully is more likely to lead to a happy sex life than to problems.

See also Sexual problems (p. 72)

MENARCHE

The onset of menstruation. Usually starts between the ages of ten and sixteen years of age.

MENOPAUSE

Most women reach the menopause between the ages of about forty and fifty-five. Their glands slow down the production of sex hormones, their ovaries stop producing eggs and their periods cease. They are no longer likely to get pregnant.

The problems that are commonly associated with the menopause are largely caused by the fall in oestrogen levels. The symptoms produced at this time include (roughly in order of frequency):

1 Hot flushes and sweats.

2 Anxiety, depression, irritability and tiredness.

3 An inability to get to sleep at night.

4 A fall in sexual interest and some pain on intercourse.

5 Aches and pains – headaches and joint pains being commonest.

6 Hair and skin changes. The skin becomes rather dry and wrinkles become unusually apparent. The head hair becomes thin and

paradoxically hair appears where it isn't wanted – on the face for example.

7 An inability to remember things and an inability to concentrate.

8 A dry and sometimes sore vagina.

9 A general loss of confidence and a feeling of not quite being so much a woman.

10 Urinary symptoms such as incontinence.

11 A burning or strange taste in the mouth.

12 An increased incidence of broken bones.

There aren't usually any breast symptoms at all and the only change in the periods due to the menopause is their disappearance! There is a tendency to blame any symptom that affects a woman in her forties or fifties on the menopause but it is important to remember that there can be other causes both for general problems and for specific menstrual disorders.

In addition to these physical manifestations of the menopause there are, of course, a number of social and psychological problems caused by the 'change of life'. The forties and fifties are something of a crossroads for all of us. Children have usually grown up and will have either left home or be preparing to do so. Death no longer appears on the distant horizon as some unlikely visitor but is instead often uncomfortably close as friends and relatives complete their lives.

And with these mental and emotional changes accompanied by significant hormonal changes it is perhaps hardly surprising that so many women feel their femininity drifting away rather more speedily than they would have liked.

Treating the problems which so often accompany the menopause is something of a therapeutic challenge. Occasionally, of course, if specific problems are troublesome enough then specific answers can be tried. Calcium supplements will help prevent bone weaknesses producing an endless series of fractures. Oestrogen creams will help give vaginal walls more suppleness. And sometimes anti-depressant pills will be needed.

But the treatment most commonly used with success is Hormone Replacement Therapy – in which a combination of oestrogen and progestogen is given orally. Although women with circulatory disorders, breast cancer, liver problems and various other diseases cannot use hormone replacement therapy (in case their symptoms are made worse) the treatment seems to be both safe and extremely effective.

Hormone replacement therapy doesn't increase a woman's chances of developing cancer, it doesn't increase her fertility and it doesn't act as a contraceptive! It does produce some mild side effects, such as breast tenderness and occasionally nausea, and it can sometimes produce unexpected menstrual bleeding.

On the other hand hormone therapy can make skin firmer, the vagina softer and moister and the whole body feel better. Women who have taken hormone replacement therapy claim that they feel better, feel sexier and enjoy life much more than they do without it.

It is sometimes argued that defying nature in this way is artificial and unnatural and a number of women who would have benefited from hormones have refused to do so because they've felt that it would be in some way interfering with an entirely ordinary process. To some extent this feeling is understandable. But, without medical intervention, many of us would have died as babies. And millions use spectacles, hearing aids and walking sticks which enable them to cheat nature.

On balance most doctors seem to think that hormone replacement therapy is often a sensible and acceptable way to deal with the unpleasant, embarrassing and sometimes destructive symptoms which frequently accompany the years of the menopause. The growing number of physicians who prescribe HRT quite freely will usually allow their patients to continue with the tablets for as long as they wish. Sometimes the treatment can be stopped after a year or two. Sometimes it needs to be continued for longer.

MENORRHAGIA

Heavy periods.

See also Period problems (p. 59)

MIDSTREAM SPECIMEN

Before urine can be tested to see whether or not it contains any infection a clean, fresh and uncontaminated sample needs to be obtained. There really isn't any point in turning up at the doctor's surgery with a sample in an old pickle jar, whisky bottle or second-hand specimen container. To obtain a useful specimen follow these instructions:

1 Find a sterile bottle, preferably a bottle or container specifically designed for laboratory specimens. It should have a label for your name and for the date.

2 Wash your hands and vaginal area with plenty of warm water. Dab dry with a clean towel.

3 Remove the top from the bottle without touching the rim or the inside of the bottle.

4 Separate your labia and start to urinate.

5 When the urine stream has been going for a second or two hold the bottle in the stream and catch a decent sized sample.

6 Put the cap on the bottle and write your name and date on the label.

All this sounds ridiculously obvious and simple but if you fail to follow these instructions you are likely to obtain a contaminated (and therefore quite useless) sample.

See also Cystitis (p. 24)

MISCARRIAGE

Usually means a spontaneous, accidental or unplanned abortion.

See also Abortion (p. 1)

NON-SPECIFIC URETHRITIS

Non-specific urethritis (also known as Non-gonococcal urethritis and as NSU) sometimes produces no symptoms at all in women. When symptoms do occur they're usually a vaginal discharge and a pain on passing urine. Chlamydia often causes non-specific urethritis.

See also Sexually transmitted disease (p. 74)

OBSTETRICIAN

Doctor who specialises in looking after pregnant women both before and during childbirth.

See also Doctor (p. 29), Gynaecologist (p. 38)

OESTROGEN

The hormone that makes a woman look like a woman. It's oestrogen that produces the curves and shapes above and below a woman's waist.

ORAL SEX

Oral sex involving a mouth and the female sexual organs is known as cunnilingus. Oral sex involving a mouth and the male sexual organs is known as fellatio. There is nothing abnormal, unhealthy or dangerous about either activity.

ORGASM

There are great mysteries and many myths about what an orgasm is, how often a woman should have one, where it originates, whose responsibility it is to see that an orgasm is obtained and so on. Those mysteries and myths have been devised and spread by countless doctors, psychotherapists, sex therapists and journalists. Today the confusion is complete.

In purely clinical terms an orgasm can be defined as a peak of sexual arousal which consists of uncontrollable muscle movements, a feeling of warmth, a tingling and an indescribable sense of joy and pleasure. Usually produced by stimulation of the clitoris (which may in turn be activated by intercourse, manual stimulation or masturbation) a failure to have an orgasm may be a result of the fact that the clitoris has not been properly stimulated or may be due to inhibitions produced by fear, anxiety or simple, old-fashioned guilt.

Although there is much confusion about just how orgasms develop, and how many women enjoy how many how often, we do know that it doesn't really matter whether an orgasm is produced by clitoral stimulation, vaginal penetration or breast fondling. There aren't several types of orgasm, there is only one. And an orgasm is an orgasm is an orgasm!

See also Clitoris (p. 20), G spot (p. 36)

OVARIES

Every normal, healthy woman has two ovaries. They are plum-sized and they have two main functions.

1 Each ovary contains tens of thousands of egg cells and every month one of those eggs must be released for possible fertilisation.

2 Ovaries also have the responsibility of producing sex hormones oestrogen and progesterone. These two hormones affect the whole of the body's growth and development as well as affecting behaviour too. It's the sex hormones which give a woman her shape and her curves. The production of oestrogen is at its peak before ovulation. After ovulation the ovaries produce both oestrogen and progesterone.

See also Anatomy (p. 6), Ovulation (p. 56)

OVULATION

When an egg is released from an ovary there is sometimes pain and bleeding. This mid-cycle pain is known as mittelschmerz pain. To stop the pain it is necessary to stop the ovulation – and a hormone pill is usually needed.

A woman who gets pain or bleeding in the middle of her cycle is probaby ovulating and is, therefore, unlikely to be infertile.

PV

Medical shorthand for a vaginal examination.

PAIN

Pain is undeniably traumatic and invariably a nuisance. But it is also a message. It is your body's way of telling you that something is wrong. Pain tells you to move when you are in danger and to rest when your body is under too much stress. Touch something hot and your body's pain perceptors will ensure that you move away quickly. Sit on a pin and you'll jump up out of the way. Pain, it is important to remember, always means something. And the more that you, and your doctor, can find out about a pain the greater your chances of finding out what is causing it and then dealing with it effectively and permanently.

So, for example, decide whether your pain is related to your menstrual periods or not. If it isn't then it may be caused by a non-gynaecological problem such as diverticulitis, appendicitis, or cystitis. If it is related to intercourse then it may be due to cervicitis, an imperforate hymen or a vaginal problem. If it is a mid-cycle pain then it may be caused by ovulation – particularly if the pain is on one side of your abdomen. If the pain is accompanied by a fever then there could be an infection somewhere. If the pain accompanies a period then it could be due to endometriosis or fibroids. If you haven't had a period for some time then the pain could be due to an ectopic pregnancy or an early abortion. If an ovarian cyst has already been found then that could have twisted or ruptured.

Don't bravely put up with persistent pain or recurrent pain. And don't use remedies you've bought yourself for more than five days. The best way to deal with pain is to find the cause – and deal with that.

PELVIC FLOOR EXERCISES

Any woman who has ever had a baby will have put her pelvic and vaginal muscles under a considerable strain. The muscles will have had to stretch to allow the baby through, and they will have had to exert pressure while being stretched. All things considered it is perhaps hardly surprising that the muscles in this region often lose their tone and strength.

Many problems can develop because of loose and flabby muscles in and around the vaginal walls. Stress incontinence, prolapses and unsatisfying sexual intercourse are just three of the most important problems. These disorders can, of course, be treated by surgery or by the use of a ring pessary but they can often be ameliorated or prevented by deliberate exercising of the muscles involved.

The muscles that control the vaginal walls also control the flow of urine from the bladder and this link can be used to advantage. So, for example, a woman wanting to strengthen her vaginal muscles should sit on the lavatory with her legs apart and her arms resting on her thighs. She should then first force a little urine out and then almost immediately use the muscles between the tops of her thighs to stop the flow.

For the next few minutes she should continue to pass teaspoonfuls of urine in bursts, contracting her muscles to control the flow.

After practising like this for a while she will be able to contract and relax the relevant muscles without needing to pass urine. And then she will be able to practise the exercise whatever else she is doing and wherever she is: at home or at work, in a supermarket queue or in a traffic jam. Once she has got quite good at it she can try putting a finger into her vagina and squeezing. She should then be able to feel her new muscle power.

Eventually, she will be able to use that muscle power to squeeze anything that happens to be inside.

See also Incontinence (p. 43), Prolapse (p. 67)

PELVIC INFLAMMATORY DISEASE

Inflammation and infection involving the tissues in the pelvis. Pelvic inflammatory disease is a fairly common cause of infertility.

See also Infertility (p. 44)

PERIODS

Every month the womb lining builds up ready to receive a fertilised egg. The growth of the lining, or endometrium, is governed by hormones produced by the ovaries. If sperm get into the womb at or around the time of ovulation and an egg is fertilised then the lining will remain where it is. If no egg is fertilised then the cells of the lining will be discharged from the womb ready for a whole new cycle of events to begin.

The discharge of the womb lining makes up the contents of a woman's monthly period.

The length of the average cycle (from the start of one period to the start of the next) is twenty-eight days but anything between twenty-one and forty-two days can be regarded as normal. The important thing is not so much the length of the cycle but its regularity. If a woman regularly has a thirty-five-day cycle then that is normal for her.

The period itself, or bleeding phase, usually lasts for between two and seven days. The average bleed lasts for four or five days. Again it is the pattern and regularity that is important. So, when a woman normally has a six-day period then a three-day period will be abnormal for her. And when a woman normally has a three-day period a six-day period will be abnormal.

PERIOD PROBLEMS

Period problems fall into four main categories: absent periods, heavy periods, irregular periods and painful periods.

Absent periods (amenorrhoea)

Periods normally begin when pituitary and ovarian hormones stimulate ovulation and menstruation. The failure of periods to start spontaneously by the age of sixteen is known as primary amenorrhoea while the failure of periods to appear after they've started normally is known as secondary amenorrhoea.

The absence of menstrual periods doesn't always mean that there is something wrong, of course. Young girls who haven't yet reached puberty don't have periods and women who have passed through the menopause don't have periods either. During pregnancy, when a fertilised egg has settled on the endometrium, there won't be any periods. After pregnancy two out of three women who breast-feed still haven't started having their periods again by the time their baby is three months old.

When there isn't a straightforward explanation for the absence of periods there can be a number of possible reasons for a woman not having a monthly bleed. Taking the contraceptive pill can cause periods to disappear – both while it is being taken and afterwards – as can other drugs and a variety of hormone problems. Stress, worry, excess dieting and anorexia nervosa can all mean that a woman doesn't have a period when she expects one.

Heavy periods (menorrhagia)

Most women lose less than 80 mls of blood a month. That's about three ounces. In practical terms that means that an average sort of woman will use about twelve tampons during a period – with about four tampons being used on the heaviest day.

Sometimes, of course, the amount of blood lost is much greater. A woman is said to have menorrhagia if she needs to use more than twenty tampons during a period (or more than about eight during one day of a period). The precise amount of blood lost during a heavy period can be measured by collecting together all the tampons in a plastic bag and then soaking them in a special solution. Heavy bleeding is sometimes accompanied by clots too and although these are rather frightening they don't usually signify anything other than a fairly severe loss.

Heavy periods can be caused in a variety of ways. Sometimes the excess blood is produced by a simple amplification of normal mechanisms, with hormone changes being responsible. Sometimes, however, an excess bleed can be caused by inflammatory disease, fibroids, an incomplete abortion, an intra-uterine contraceptive device or even a clotting disorder. When a bleed is particularly heavy, and the problem persists for month after month, the commonest side effect is anaemia. The main symptoms of anaemia are pallor, tiredness and breathlessness.

Before menorrhagia can be treated it is, of course, necessary to try and find a cause. One of the commonest diagnostic methods used is a D & C (dilatation and curettage). Once a diagnosis has been established treatment can begin. If there is a specific problem such as fibroids or inflammatory disease then the treatment will be relatively straightforward. If it's a clotting disorder then a drug may be needed. If the bleeding is being caused by a prostaglandin problem then a prostaglandin synthetase inhibitor, usually a non-steroidal anti-inflammatory agent such as indomethacin or mefanamic acid, may be needed. Sometimes a drug called Danazol is used to inhibit pituitary hormones. Occasionally hormone pills may help. And from time to time a hysterectomy may be the only answer.

The important thing to remember is that heavy periods need investigating and can usually be treated.

Irregular periods

Irregular periods always need investigating. They can be caused by an ectopic pregnancy, any sort of abortion, a lesion affecting the cervix, a hormonal problem, a polyp, an intra-uterine contraceptive device and a dozen other things. Infertility is sometimes an associated problem since a woman who has irregular periods may not be ovulating. Anovulatory periods are particularly likely during adolescence, after an abortion, after childbirth and during the menopause. The solution depends on the cause but the contraceptive pill is often the answer.

Painful periods (dysmenorrhoea)

Period pains are usually divided into two groups: those which start a year or two after puberty (known as primary dysmenorrhoea) and those which start after years of painless menstruation (known as secondary dysmenorrhoea).

The onset of pain in primary dysmenorrhoea usually comes at about the time when ovulation starts, and it is caused by the uterine contractions which the production of prostaglandins has inspired. It's a colicky sort of pain, coming a few hours before menstruation, lasting for about a day and sometimes being accompanied by nausea, sweating, fainting and constipation. The pain is usually situated in the lower part of the abdomen, and it usually goes into the thighs and lower part of the buttocks. Two thirds of the girls who develop primary dysmenorrhoea have a family history of such pains and it is quite likely that many girls who get pains do so because they have been warned by their mothers to expect a lot of suffering. The power of the mind over the body can be considerable, and someone expecting pain usually gets it. That doesn't mean, of course, that primary dysmenorrhoea isn't real enough at the time and it certainly needs sympathy and treatment. Over the counter remedies are usually pretty useless and fairly ineffective but the pain can usually be controlled either by giving a contraceptive pill for a few months to suppress ovulation or by giving an anti-prostaglandin such as indomethacin or mefanamic acid to control the prostaglandin production. The best, simple, painkillers, for use when the pain is at its worst, are aspirin and paracetamol.

Secondary dysmenorrhoea can be produced in a number of different ways. It always (by definition) develops after years of pain-free menstruation and can be caused by infections, endometriosis, pelvic inflammatory disease, fibroids, polyps, cancer, intra-uterine contraceptive devices, bowel disorders, skeletal problems, urinary disorders and just about anything else you care to think of! Finding the right treatment for secondary dysmenorrhoea naturally depends on finding the cause of the pain.

PILLS (CONTRACEPTIVE)

Millions of women around the world currently use the contraceptive pill, and scores of different brands are available. There are some risks and side effects associated with the contraceptive pill's use, of course, but the dangers have undoubtedly been over-emphasised by newspaper reporters looking for 'scare' stories and by religious campaigners trying to oppose a form of contraception which has undoubtedly been a major cause of sexual permissiveness. Although it is still necessary to ensure that those women who are especially at risk avoid taking the pill there is now a good deal of solid research to show that the risks associated with being pregnant are considerably greater than the risks of taking the contraceptive pill. Avoiding sex altogether would undoubtedly be safer still but that isn't an option many people are prepared to consider.

Although there are, as I've already pointed out, scores of different brands of contraceptive pill there are only three main types of pill available. These are the combined pill, the progestogen-only pill and the triphasic pill.

The combined pill

This is the contraceptive pill most widely prescribed. It contains a mixture of oestrogen and progestogen. It stops the ovaries producing their own hormones and therefore stops ovulation. It also changes the womb lining so that any egg which did manage to get out and get fertilised wouldn't stand much of a chance of getting properly embedded. The combined pill also thickens the cervical mucus and makes it more difficult for sperm to get into the uterus.

The very many different types of combined pill often contain slightly different proportions of oestrogen and progestogen; consequently the side effects associated with the different pills also vary. Problems which have been reported with contraceptive pills include: acne, weight gain, migraine, sore breasts, swollen legs, vaginal discharge, nausea, headache, depression, spotting or breakthrough bleeding, and a high blood pressure. In a very small number of women clots have formed, sometimes causing strokes and even death.

When one or two side effects are particularly troublesome it is sometimes possible to deal with the problems simply by changing the pill. To avoid the more serious, potentially damaging hazards it is probably sensible not to take a combined pill if you have a family or personal history of circulatory disease, if you are over thirty-five years of age or if you are a moderate to heavy smoker. Having said that I must admit that the risks of taking a contraceptive pill are probably still comparable with or less than the risks associated with pregnancy or abortion.

Most combined pills need to be taken once a day for twenty-one days. They are then left off for seven days, during which time a withdrawal bleed occurs.

The progestogen-only pill (mini pill)

As its name suggests this pill contains only progestogen. It's safer than the combined pill in many respects and it can often be used by women who can't take that. It works by altering the lining of the womb and by thickening the mucus at the cervix and is slightly less efficient than the combined pill.

The progestogen-only pill is usually taken without a break.

The triphasic pill

This relatively new innovation contains variable doses of oestrogen and progestogen and is said to have fewer side effects. It seems both safe and acceptable but is not yet as widely available or as well tried as the ordinary combined pill.

Those, then, are the three main types of contraceptive pill which are available. Anyone taking a hormonal contraceptive should remember that periods are usually scanty – and may even disappear altogether – while a pill is being taken. It is also important to remember that contraceptive pills don't always mix well with other tablets and medicines. So, for example, some antibiotics and painkillers may nullify the effect of the contraceptive pill. If you're taking the contraceptive pill don't take an over the counter medicine. And if you're given a prescription for another drug by a doctor tell him you're on the pill and ask whether you should take additional precautions.

After a contraceptive pill has been stopped menstrual periods may be erratic for a month or two. Ovulation may be only occasional too. There are probably not any risks in a woman conceiving immediately after stopping the contraceptive pill but my own feeling is that women should stop their pills six months before they intend to get pregnant and that they should use other

63

precautions for that time – just to avoid any possible risks to their baby.

See also Contraception (p. 22)

POLYPS

A smooth lump on a stalk that projects into the centre of a hollow organ. Polyps fairly commonly exist inside the uterus. They can cause a discharge or irregular bleeding and they can be diagnosed and treated by curettage.

POST-COITAL CONTRACEPTION

Two pills of ethinyloestradiol taken within seventy-two hours of intercourse and followed by two pills of the same substance twelve hours later will prevent a woman getting pregnant, by preventing implantation should an egg have been fertilised.

This method seems both safe and effective and is recommended for just about all women. It has few, if any, side effects and there doesn't seem to be any reason why it shouldn't be used as a routine method of contraception for those who enjoy occasional or unexpected intercourse. Because the hormone doses used are relatively low (four pills are used in a fairly short time but these are similar pills to ones used in the preparation of normal contra-ceptives) there shouldn't be any of the difficulties often experienced with contraceptive pills.

Morning-after pills can only be used up to seventy-two hours after sex but copper intra-uterine contraceptive devices, inserted up to five days after sex, also have a contraceptive effect after the event and these are clearly suitable for women who haven't been able to seek medical advice within the seventy-two-hour period.

Incidentally, the record for the shortest time interval between sex and post-coital contraception seems to be held at ten minutes. A boyfriend is reported as having turned up, breathless, at a doctor's surgery just ten minutes after discovering that his condom had split while in use!

See also Contraception (p. 22)

PRE-MENSTRUAL SYNDROME

Something like fifty per cent of all women suffer uncomfortable, painful and annoying symptoms before their periods. Half of those suffer badly. The symptoms associated with the pre-menstrual syndrome vary a good deal but include: depression, irritability, tension, headaches, an inability to concentrate, gastro-intestinal symptoms such as indigestion, diarrhoea and constipation, breast tenderness, fluid retention, palpitations, a change in sexual interest (either for the better or for the worse), faintness, dizziness, an inability to cope with extremes of heat or cold, changes in eating habits, an inability to get to sleep at night and palpitations. Diseases such as asthma, migraine and eczema get worse during the time immediately prior to a period and stress-induced problems all deteriorate. Because of the mental changes which take place many women report that problems at work, at home or with the law have got worse because of incidents taking place before a period is due.

The importance of the pre-menstrual syndrome has become clearer in recent years for several reasons. First, of course, there has been an increase in general awareness of the existence of the problem. Second, there has been an increase in the number of women doctors (and therefore an increase in pressure on the medical profession to recognise the problem as a real disorder and not just a little difficulty affecting women). Third, the modern woman has far more periods than her ancestors. Today's woman lives to seventy and has, on average, just two children. If she menstruates from the age of fifteen to the age of forty-five she'll have to put up with a total of about 400 monthly periods. Yesterday's woman had more children, breast-fed more often and had fewer periods.

Diagnosing the pre-menstrual syndrome can sometimes be tricky. There has, in recent years, been a tendency for sufferers and doctors to blame all problems affecting women on 'the time of the month'. In practice, however, the diagnosis can be made with some certainty if care is taken to make sure that all the symptoms thought to be associated with the onset of the periods are truly cyclical (they come, get worse and go, come, get worse and go, etc.). When the symptoms don't get better or disappear altogether after a monthly period they are unlikely to be anything to do with the pre-menstrual syndrome. Any woman who is uncertain about whether or not particular problems are linked to her periods should simply keep a daily chart, showing when the symptoms appear, when they get worse, and when they go away.

There is still a good deal of confusion about the best way to treat the pre-menstrual syndrome. Some experts believe that the best solution is to prescribe progesterone while others claim that most sufferers have normal progesterone levels. Some women have enjoyed considerable relief from symptoms by using vitamin B6 (pyridoxine). In doses up to 100 mg twice a day pyridoxine seems to have an effect on both the pituitary gland and the ovaries.

Sometimes more specific solutions can be tried. So, for example, women who swell up a good deal will sometimes benefit from using diuretics to help them get rid of fluid. Overweight women sometimes feel better after dieting. Women who get a lot of pain obtain relief from prostaglandin synthetase inhibitors such as indomethacin or mefanamic acid.

Keeping the blood sugar up by eating regular meals seems to help some. Avoiding salt, caffeine and alcohol during the days before a period helps others. Breast symptoms can occasionally be relieved by using bromocriptine. Evening primrose oil capsules are being used with considerable success by some experts. If depression becomes severe drug therapy may be needed and if anxiety is disabling the very short-term use of tranquillisers may be acceptable. Danazol is sometimes used to suppress pituitary hormones while the ordinary contraceptive pill is also sometimes prescribed as a solution.

Remedies bought over the counter, on the other hand, rarely seem successful and apart from aspirin and paracetamol (still the best remedies for pain) and pyridoxine (which really ought to be used under a doctor's supervision) I don't know of anything you can buy without a prescription which I would recommend.

Finally it is important not only that the sufferer herself understands the problems associated with the pre-menstrual syndrome but that her husband or boyfriend understands too. Understanding the problem doesn't solve anything but it does sometimes make it easier to bear.

PROGESTERONE

Hormone which has the job of preparing the uterus for the implantation of an embryo – and also for maintaining a pregnancy once it has developed. A progestogen is a compound that has a progesterone-like quality.

PROLAPSE

Normally the uterus sits in the abdomen with only the cervix projecting down into the upper part of the vagina. The womb is kept in position by a network of muscles and ligaments. Sometimes, however, the supports become weakened and the womb falls down and into the vagina. Technically there are three stages for a prolapse:

1 In a first degree prolapse the womb falls down but stays inside the vagina.

2 In a second degree prolapse the womb stays inside the vagina for most of the time but if the sufferer coughs or sneezes it will pop outside through the vestibule. This can be frightening and startling – for the cervix will be clearly visible.

3 In a third degree prolapse the muscles which support the womb are so weak that the womb and cervix remain hanging through the vestibule all the time. When this happens the prolapsed womb is known as a procidentia and the main risk is that chafing will cause bleeding and a considerable amount of soreness. The vaginal walls actually get turned inside out too so that they are hanging outside the vulva.

Those are the three basic types of prolapse. In addition weaknesses of the tissues in and around the vagina can also produce an urethrocele (a prolapse of the urethra) a cystocele (a prolapse of the bladder) and a rectocele (a prolapse of the rectum).

Since all these problems are caused by a stretching and weakening of the muscles and ligaments which normally hold all these organs in place it is hardly surprising that prolapses of all kinds are commonest among women who have had a number of children. Prolapses are particularly likely to occur when labours have been long and difficult. Other factors which affect the likelihood of a prolapse developing are the menopause (which affects the

67

production of natural hormones), obesity (which puts a straight-forward physical strain on the tissues) heavy lifting (which strains and weakens muscles) and coughing (which increases the pressure inside the abdomen and therefore helps to push the uterus out of the vagina).

An overweight woman of fifty-five who has three children, who smokes regularly and who coughs every morning will be a prime candidate for a prolapse.

There are several ways in which a prolapse can be tackled. If the muscle weakness is relatively slight then pelvic floor exercises, designed to strengthen the muscles, may help. Alternatively a ring pessary (designed to hold the womb in place) may be a suitable answer. If a pessary is put in by the way it is important to remember to change it every six months or so. Left in place for too long pessaries can cause inflammation and infection.

If, however, the prolapse is severe and the muscle weakness considerable an operation will probably be needed to repair the tissues and re-sling the organs involved. Sometimes, when a prolapse is accompanied by other symptoms for example, a hysterectomy may be the only sensible solution.

See also Anatomy (p. 6), Incontinence (p. 43), Pelvic floor exercises (p. 57), Uterus (p. 82)

PROSTAGLANDINS

Prostaglandins are powerful, internally produced drugs which are not stored but which are made at the site where they are needed and are then used more or less straightaway. They were first thought to be secreted only by the prostate gland in the male (that's where they got their name from) but were later found to be produced in many different parts of the human body – in both men and women – and to have a variety of separate actions.

One of the effects that prostaglandins have in women is to stimulate uterine muscles to contract. They also have some effect on the menstrual cycle. Although there is still much mystery about precisely how prostaglandins work we do know that their actions can be effectively opposed by the use of 'inhibiting' drugs such as indomethacin and mefanamic acid.

PUBERTY

The age at which girls stop being girls and start being women is changing generation by generation. A century or so ago girls used to reach the onset of puberty at the age of fourteen or fifteen. Today girls are beginning to show all the early signs of puberty – sprouting breasts, thighs that flare, strands of pubic hair and menstrual periods – at twelve, eleven and even ten years of age. We can probably thank general, fairly dramatic improvements in living conditions for this.

Puberty starts when the hypothalamus (a part of the brain) stimulates the pituitary gland. The pituitary gland, in turn, produces hormones which stimulate the ovary and the ovary then releases an egg. If the egg is fertilised a baby will be produced. If the egg isn't fertilised it will be discharged, together with the womb lining, as a menstrual period.

Puberty can be considered a problem if it starts before the age of eight (the world record is held by a girl who started her periods at the age of eight months and by the age of just over five and a half years was a mother herself). When that happens it is usually due to some constitutional problem. And it's often something that runs in the family. At the other end of the age spectrum puberty is also a problem if it still hasn't arrived by the time a girl reaches the age of sixteen. There may be nothing to worry about, of course. But it is worth getting a medical opinion, nevertheless.

PUBIC HAIR

Pubic hair highlights the pubic area, provides some protection and helps to retain the sexually stimulating secretions which are produced locally. Developing at puberty as a few wispy strands of hair along the labia, pubic hair spreads upwards over the pubis, then covers the mons too.

Normally pubic hair in women doesn't spread on to the thighs and nor does it spread upwards across the lower part of the abdomen as it does in men. There is usually a fairly straight upper edge to the pubic hair so that a fairly neat triangle is produced.

When pubic hair does spread outwards on to the thighs or upwards towards the umbilicus there is usually some hormonal imbalance and these outward signs are often accompanied by problems such as amenorrhoea and infertility. Hormone-containing pills can be used to deal with the problem in most cases.

RETROVERSION

Under normal circumstances the uterus is bent slightly forward, resting on the bladder and lying at an angle of ninety degrees to the vagina. Sometimes, however, the uterus is bent backwards – this is known as retroversion.

Retroversion isn't particularly important nor is it dangerous but some doctors think it can cause backache and may make it difficult for a woman to conceive.

See also Uterus (p. 82)

RHYTHM METHOD

Both the male sperm and the female egg can survive for no more than a few days. For fertilisation to take place, and pregnancy to ensue, the sperm and the egg must be in roughly the same place at roughly the same time. Since the egg is released at ovulation, which normally takes place roughly midway between menstrual cycles, it is possible to estimate just when conception is most likely to take place. The same information naturally makes it possible to estimate when conception is least likely to take place. That is the principle behind the rhythm method.

An egg can live for about two days and sperm have a potential life span of about the same length. Theoretically, that means that if sperm can be kept out of the vagina for two days each side of ovulation then the woman is unlikely to get pregnant.

The key to this form of contraception is, of course, the time of ovulation. This is normally thought to take place about fourteen days before the beginning of a menstrual period and so those who believe in the merits of the rhythm method usually suggest that intercourse is avoided between the tenth and twentieth days of the cycle – as long as the cycle is regular.

In order to give the rhythm method more of a scientific sound to it some exponents try to measure the moment of ovulation by measuring body temperature. It is thought that the body temperature of a woman goes down slightly and then up slightly when an egg is released. So daily temperature readings will, theoretically at least, help the two partners avoid that time of the cycle more efficiently.

A variation on this theme, known as the Billings Method, depends on the fact that the mucus in the vagina becomes slightly less sticky at this crucial time of the month. This form of contraception naturally depends on the ability of the female partner (or even her consort) to assess the stickiness of her vaginal mucus.

All these forms of contraception depend on the periods being regular and on ovulation occurring more or less when expected. If the periods are not regular or if ovulation is unpredictable then the method is not a good one.

Although they can hardly be described as 'natural' these rhythm methods are popular in some parts of the world with those who, following strong religious convictions, disapprove of barrier or hormonal methods of contraception.

Family planning experts claim that they have a word to describe those individuals who practise the rhythm method. They call them 'parents'.

See also Contraception (p. 22)

RING PESSARY

To keep a prolapsed uterus in position a ring shaped piece of plastic, glass or metal is sometimes used. When a ring pessary is used it should be taken out and replaced every six months or so if infection is to be avoided.

See also Prolapse (p. 67)

SCABIES

The main symptoms of scabies is itching – particularly at night. It's a disease that is easily passed around within a family and since it is often passed from one sexual partner to another it can be classed as a sexually transmitted disease. Tell-tale burrows can sometimes be found in the skin but the commonest signs are the superficial scratches produced by the sufferers own nails!

Scabies can be treated with either 10 per cent benzoyl benzoate or 1 per cent gamma benzene hydrochloride. The lotion should be applied to all areas of the body that are affected and should be left there for twenty-four hours before being washed off in the bath. Clothes and bedclothes should be laundered too.

See also Sexually transmitted diseases (p. 74)

SEX DETERMINATION

It is possible to have tests done which will show the sex of an unborn baby. However, the only point in having such a test done is to abort any baby of an unwanted sex. And such a procedure is still illegal in most parts of the world. Were it to be made legal the social consequences would be disastrous.

I know of no trick guaranteed to provide a child of selected sex.

SEXUAL PROBLEMS

It's difficult to categorise sexual problems; there are probably as many causes and explanations as there are individuals with difficulties. The majority of sexual problems affecting women do, however, fall into the following groups:

Problems caused by pain

Only a confirmed masochist enjoys sex when it hurts – and there are lots of reasons why it can hurt. Superficial pains and soreness can be caused by vaginal dryness, by localised infections, by allergy reactions and by cuts or sores. Forgotten tampons, and other objects, left inside the vagina can cause considerable discomfort, and cystitis is another source of distress. A rigid hymen, an opening made too small after an episiotomy and old scarring can also cause problems.

Deeper pains can be caused by endometriosis, ovarian cysts, fibroids, chronic pelvic congestion (sometimes produced by having intercourse repeatedly and constantly failing to reach an orgasm) a retroverted uterus, an infection of the cervix or a prolapse. In all those cases the sexual problem will only be resolved when the underlying disorder is treated.

Problems caused by fear, guilt, etc.

A woman who is frightened of getting pregnant or frightened of contracting a sexually transmitted disease won't enjoy sex. She'll be tense and 'tight' and sex will probably be uncomfortable and unpleasant.

Guilt is another common cause of unhappy, unsatisfying sex. A woman who feels bad about a relationship, or who is frightened of being discovered in a compromising situation isn't likely to enjoy the experience. It's difficult to reach an orgasm if you're constantly waiting for the living room door to open or for someone to tap on the car window and shine a torch into your face. Many of those who suffer most from guilt do so because they have been brought up to think of sex as something rather 'dirty' and 'unnatural'.

Problems caused by disinterest

If you're not really interested in sex and you're only doing it because it seems the decent thing to do then you're not likely to get much pleasure out of it! It is important to be aware that although a lack of interest in sex is often due to the fact that there is no love or even life left in a relationship a loss of libido may be due to drugs and pills of many kinds. The contraceptive pill can adversely affect sexual interest and so can many widely used tranquillisers and sleeping tablets. The benzodiazepines, for example, can have a very negative effect on sexual feelings.

Male problems

Sounds obvious but if he is impotent or if he ejaculates prematurely then she isn't going to get much pleasure out of sex.

A high proportion of women who think they have sexual problems are suffering from nothing more (or less) than a man who is either incapable of performing properly or too selfish to ensure that his partner gets as much satisfaction as he does.

SEXUALLY TRANSMITTED DISEASES

There are more than twenty-five different types of sexually transmitted disease although if you counted all the diseases that *could* be transmitted from one sexual partner to another you'd have to include impetigo, measles, and the common cold so the list could be as long as the proverbial piece of string.

The incidence of sexually transmitted disease has been rising steadily for the last few decades. It goes up by between five per cent and ten per cent every year. In Britain alone there are now about half a million cases a year – and that is not counting those patients who go to see their own general practitioner, those who see gynaecologists and those who see private doctors. The half a million figure refers only to those individuals seen in the so-called 'special' clinics at British hospitals. STDs are among the most common diseases in the world.

Sexually transmitted diseases are caused by bacteria, parasites, yeasts, viruses, chlamydiae, fungi, and mites. The symptoms include rashes, swellings, urinary symptoms (such as bleeding, frequency and pain), soreness, itching, discharges that have increased, changed or become smelly, lumps, ulcers and warts. Bleeding and pain are another couple of common presenting problems.

The picture is confused by the fact that sexually transmitted diseases are often passed on in surprise bundles – with contacts handing over several different infections at once – and that many sufferers don't have any symptoms at all.

Reliable statistics are difficult to come by but the commonest sexually transmitted diseases are probably candida, trichomonas, non-specific urethritis, gonorrhoea, warts and herpes. The three symptoms to look out for are sores, ulcers and a discharge.

Once a sexually transmitted disease has been caught it must be diagnosed and treated just as quickly as possible. And that means a visit to a doctor, hospital or clinic. The complications that can be caused are numerous and can be very damaging. Pelvic infections and inflammatory diseases are among the most serious problems but women with STDs who get pregnant are likely to infect their babies too. On the whole women seem more likely to suffer serious problems from STDs than men, perhaps because they are less likely to notice symptoms at an early stage and therefore less likely to obtain early and effective treatment.

Avoiding a sexually transmitted disease is something of a problem. It isn't easy to spot sufferers (and signs and symptoms may not be apparent even on fairly close examination). Mechanical forms of contraception such as condoms, diaphragms and even spermicidal creams seem to provide some protection and you can probably help a little by passing urine after sex and by washing yourself with soap and water too.

The best advice I can give is that if you even *suspect* that you could have a sexually transmitted disease go and get professional advice just as soon as possible.

SPERMICIDES

Chemicals – available in creams, pessaries, tablets, foams, aerosols, etc. – which kill sperm. They are messy and need to be used together with other forms of contraceptive protection since they are fairly ineffective.

(See also Contraception (p. 22)

STERILISATION

More and more women who decide that they have enough children are opting for sterilisation. After all, if you're thirty-five and you've got two children then you're probably going to have another ten years during which you'll have to take contraceptive pre-cautions. That's probably too long to keep on taking the pill and its a long time to have to rely on other forms of contraception.

Several types of sterilisation operation are performed but in the quickest, simplest and commonest the gynaecologist simply makes a small hole in the abdomen (either a laparotomy or a laparoscopy) and then attacks the Fallopian tubes. He will either cut and remove part of the tubes, seal them with clips or rings or seal them shut with diathermy. The whole procedure takes no more than twenty minutes and it usually involves no more than one or perhaps two days in hospital. Since there is now no way for eggs to reach the uterus, pregnancy is effectively prevented.

Sometimes, when other problems exist and there are other symptoms to be considered a gynaecologist will remove the whole of the womb or the womb AND the ovaries. This is a rather more drastic operation and it will involve a longer stay in hospital; it is only done when the need for sterilistion is accompanied by other problems such as fibroids, heavy bleeding or some severe inflammatory disease.

If a sterilisation operation is done properly there will be very little chance of the woman ever getting pregnant again. It is always difficult to be certain about anything in medicine and very occasionally Fallopian tubes do grow together again. But, by and large, a sterilisation operation puts an end to a woman's reproductive years. Reversing the operation is occasionally possible but it is difficult and unreliable.

After a sterilisation a woman will notice little if any difference. Her hormone production won't stop (unless her ovaries have also been removed) and her sex life is likely to be improved because the fear of conception will have disappeared. The only women who do suffer are the ones who were not certain about sterilisation in the first place. Any woman who contemplates sterilisation as a serious solution to her long-term contraception problem should be aware that it means that she will never have any more children. A woman who finds this a cheering thought is probably a good candidate for sterilisation. A woman who finds it a daunting or frightening thought should probably think again.

The sterilisation operation does provide immediate cover in that it stops any more eggs getting into the womb but it is wise to take additional precautions until the next menstrual period. There is always the risk that an egg may have already got into the womb and be waiting to be fertilised.

So far I have dealt only with female sterilisation. It is, of course, also possible for men to be sterilised. This is an extremely simple operation which involves cutting the two tubes or vas deferens through which sperm pass from the testes to the penis. When the tubes are cut sperm cannot get into the ejaculate and although there are no visible differences afterwards a man will be sterile after ten or twenty ejaculations have cleared waiting sperm from the near side part of the two tubes. Men are usually advised to have two tests done afterwards to check that their semen no longer contains sperm.

The male sterilisation operation takes only ten or twenty minutes and can be done under a local anaesthetic. Like the female sterilisation operation it is one that should be regarded as a permanent solution. The operation can sometimes be reversed but it is a tricky and unreliable procedure.

See also Contraception (p. 22)

STRETCH MARKS

When you were born you probably weighed about seven pounds. Today you probably weigh about twenty times as much. As your body has grown so your skin will have stretched and adapted to contain the increasing mass of bone, muscle and so on. If your skin had not stretched you would have burst out of it long ago.

Human skin can cope with these changes in weight and shape very successfully. The dermis, the deeper layer of the skin, contains a number of elastic fibres and it is these which provide the skin with its elastic qualities. These fibres do, however, need time to do their job properly. When changes are made rapidly the skin doesn't adapt anywhere near so successfully and stretch marks commonly appear – their number and size being roughly proportional to the rate of weight change.

In simple mechanical terms the skin is stretched too quickly and the elastic fibres are permanently damaged.

There are other reasons for the development of stretch marks too. It is now known that hormonal changes can also play an important part in stretch mark formation and it seems that some hormones (in particular one called cortisone that is produced by the suprarenal glands) weaken and rupture the elastic fibres in the dermis while mechanical forces subsequently decide the extent, length, site and direction of the marks.

Stretch marks usually appear first during adolescence when there is often a change in hormone levels in the body. Girls are twice as likely as boys to develop marks, or striae as they are also known, but about a third of all teenagers suffer from them. Stretch marks vary in length and are usually pink or purple to begin with and only turn white later. The commonest site for stretch marks is probably on the abdomen although some girls also get them on their breasts – particularly when the development there is considerable. Obviously the bigger the bust the greater the strain – and the greater the chance of stretch marks appearing.

The one condition that is often responsible for the development of stretch marks is pregnancy, when the female abdomen has to stretch considerably to cope with the growing baby. The result is often a host of extremely visible striae. Something like four out of five pregnant women get stretch marks (called *striae gravidarum*) and although it is the abdomen that is most commonly affected the breasts are also commonly involved since they often swell with accumulated milk.

Apart from avoiding adolescence, pregnancy and any sudden weight gain there is no certain way of ensuring that no stretch marks ever develop but some experts do claim that you can minimise the formation of striae by keeping muscles in trim and skin moist. I don't think there is anything to be gained by buying special creams – a good simple moisturising cream used in liberal quantities is probably as good as anything.

When stretch marks have developed and are a real problem the most effective (and safest) solution is probably to buy a cosmetic masking cream. Women sometimes ask about having plastic surgery for stretch marks but to be perfectly honest I don't think it's a sensible solution. It is very difficult to remove stretch marks without leaving scars which look just as bad. Masking creams are only a temporary solution but they do make marks much less apparent.

Finally, although stretch marks don't usually disappear altogether they do usually fade as the years go by.

SYPHILIS

It begins with a painless sore or chancre which looks like an ulcer and which appears on the vulva or the penis. The glands are usually up at this stage and most sufferers have a flu-like illness too. In the secondary stage, when sufferers are extremely infectious, there are skin lesions and hair loss while in the final or tertiary stage heart or brain disease is common. Syphilis can be passed from a mother to her baby (causing congenital problems) and it is, if left untreated, one of the most horrifying of the sexually transmitted diseases.

The first symptoms of syphilis can appear anything from nine to ninety days after intercourse with an infected partner and even if left untreated they usually disappear spontaneously after a few weeks or months. Sufferers stop being infectious about two years after contracting the disease although the infection can still be passed on to babies after that. The third stage isn't reached for twenty or thirty years.

Diagnosing syphilis isn't easy – particularly in women. It is important that any ulcer, however small, be investigated and tested if there is any possibility that it could be syphilitic. Caught in the early stages syphilis can be treated effectively with antibiotics such a penicillin.

See also Sexually transmitted disease (p. 74)

TAMPONS

Invented half a century ago by an American doctor whose wife got fed up with wearing bulky sanitary towels the first internal tampons were merely slightly adapted surgical tampons. Today they are widely used by millions of women who prefer them to sanitary towels because they are less bulky and less obvious and because they help to reduce the inconvenience caused by monthly menstrual bleeding.

Used properly they are neither dangerous nor uncomfortable. To avoid problems tampons with deodorants should never be used, plastic applicators should be used with extreme caution (if at all) because they can scrape and damage the inside of the vagina and super absorbent tampons should only be used when standard or regular tampons aren't capable of coping with the flow of blood. It's not a good idea to change tampons too often (because if you do the inside of the vagina can get too dry) and it is always important to remember to remove tampons (forgotten tampons are a common cause of vaginal discharge and infection).

Some women now use 'natural' sponges instead of manufactured tampons. They claim that these are more comfortable and (because they can be washed and used again) less expensive. It is, however, important to remember that natural sponges can contain impurities such as mercury and sand – they need to be washed very thoroughly before being used.

TEST-TUBE BABIES

When the Fallopian tubes are blocked eggs can't get through from the ovaries to the uterus. And that makes a woman infertile. A modern solution to this problem is to remove an egg from the ovary when it is ripe and ready to be released, to fertilise it with the father's sperm in a test tube, to allow the fertilised egg to begin to develop and to then place the early foetus directly into the mother's womb.

As long as the whole procedure is done at precisely the right moment the endometrium inside the uterus will be ready to receive the fertilised egg and the developing baby will settle in place just as it would have done if the fertilisation had been entirely natural.

See also Infertility (p. 44)

TOXIC SHOCK

This acute and dangerous illness is probably caused by an organism called staphylococcus aureus. The symptoms vary but include fever, vomiting, diarrhoea, pharyngitis, headache, conjunctivitis, rashes, swollen limbs, abdominal pains and peeling skin. Patients may also have general shock symptoms such as the sort of faintness and dizziness caused by a low blood pressure.

Back in the early 1980s toxic shock was associated specifically with the use of tampons and there was, for a while, a slight revolt against these convenient and well tried aids. A number of women and some experts believed that the use of any sort of tampon could increase the likelihood of toxic shock developing.

Today, it is thought that the bug which causes toxic shock needs rather special conditions in which to thrive and that old menstrual blood is just one of the factors involved. It has also been shown that tampons made with cellulose chips are particularly likely to encourage the growth of staphylococcus aureus (these tampons are no longer on sale) and that the scraping of the inside of the vagina with a plastic applicator can also lead to difficulties (women who use a plastic applicator should take care not to scrape away any of the vaginal lining).

If the ordinary rules of hygiene are followed and tampons are used with care there shouldn't be any problems.

TRICHOMONAS

The symptoms which accompany this infection include a yellow green vaginal discharge which often smells extremely nasty, a redness and soreness around the vagina and a tendency for sexual intercourse to be extremely painful and uncomfortable. Although trichomonas is a sexually transmitted disease it can be passed on via infected towels or infected lavatory seats too.

Since trichomonas is often present together with thrush and gonorrhoea it is often necessary for the doctor to take a vaginal swab in order to make a precise diagnosis. Once the diagnosis has been confirmed treatment will usually consist of a drug called metronidazole (which may be prescribed by a brand name). People taking this drug are usually advised not to drink any alcohol since the two don't go together very well.

Because trichomonas is a sexually transmitted disease it is often wise for the woman's partner to be treated as well.

See also Candida (p. 15), Discharge (p. 28), Sexually transmitted disease (p. 74)

ULTRASOUND

If a high pitched beam of sound – an ultrasonic beam – is passed through human tissues it will bounce back from the interfaces between tissues of different acoustic densities. By measuring exactly how far the sound beam bounces it is possible to differentiate between hollow, cystic growths and solid lumps of tissue.

Ultrasound can, therefore, be used to differentiate between ovarian cysts and muscular fibroids. It can also be used to find out exactly how many developing babies are in a womb, which way round they are and so on.

Although ultrasound is a very useful diagnostic tool it is also potentially hazardous if used unwisely or excessively. The growing baby has a very delicate hearing apparatus and unless ultrasound is used with caution that apparatus can be damaged.

URODYNAMICS

Studies of bladder and urethral function designed to help doctors assess various forms of treatment – in urodynamics the pressures and forces on urine flow are measured.

UTERUS

The uterus or womb is a hollow organ made up of very powerful muscles. The lining inside the uterus is called the endometrium and every month, under hormonal influence, this is prepared to receive and nurture a fertilised egg. If no fertilised egg settles there then the lining will be shed as a menstrual period. If an egg does settle there then it will slowly grow into a baby and as it grows so the uterus will stretch.

The part of the uterus that projects into the top part of the vagina is known as the cervix and because cancer can sometimes develop here scrapings of cells are taken for laboratory examination. The rest of the uterus is known as the body and it lies forward at an angle of about ninety per cent to the direction of the vagina. The two Fallopian tubes, one on the left and one on the right, open into the top part of the uterus.

The uterus is kept in place by a number of supporting ligaments. As the years go by these ligaments sometimes weaken (particularly if a woman has had a lot of children) and the uterus falls down into the vagina. Sometimes the prolapse that results goes far enough to appear between the labia majora.

Although the uterus is merely designed to house children things can go wrong. Fibroids can develop in the walls, endometrial tissue can appear in the wrong places (endometriosis) and cancer can develop inside the womb as well as on the cervix.

See also Anatomy (p. 6), Cancer (p. 11), Hysterectomy (p. 41), Prolapse (p. 67), Retroversion (p. 70), Ring pessary (p. 71)

VAGINA

Anatomists, who have no sense of romance, describe the vagina as a tube made of very elastic muscles and lined with a mucous membrane which is similar to the membrane lining the human mouth. Its functions are said to be allowing menstrual blood to escape from the womb, providing temporary accommodation for the male penis and offering an avenue down which a developed baby can escape from the womb.

Projecting into the innermost end of the vagina is the cervix, or neck of the womb. In virgins the outer opening of the vagina is closed by the hymen or maidenhead.

The walls of the vagina produce their own special moisturising fluid which continually passes out through the gap between the labia majora. This fluid is designed to act as an automatic, natural cleanser and to make sexual intercourse easier and more comfortable.

See also Anatomy (p. 6)

VAGINITIS

The most common symptoms of vaginitis – in inflammation of the vagina – are soreness and a discharge. Passing urine usually causes pain and sexual intercourse does too. Sometimes, when vaginitis is severe, sufferers get pain when they walk.

The commonest causes of vaginitis are candida and trichomonas infections and effective treatment naturally requires a precise diagnosis. Since both these infections can be transmitted by sexual intercourse it is important for a woman's sexual partner to be treated too. While treatment is being carried out it is best to avoid sex completely – or for the male to use a sheath contraceptive.

VENEREAL DISEASE

See Sexually transmitted disease (p. 74)

VULVAL PROBLEMS

The vulva can be affected by direct infections (such as candida, trichomonas, chlamydia, herpes, gonorrhoea, etc.) or by secondary infections accompanying problems such as obesity, scratched or cut skin, incontinence, urinary problems, prolapse or a vaginal discharge. The skin around the vulva can be affected by eczema and psoriasis and swellings in, on or around the vulva may be caused by genital warts, sebaceous cysts, abscesses of Bartholin's glands or simply fatty lumps. Remnants of a torn hymen may hang around the vulva and general disorders such as diabetes can cause localised infections to develop. Threadworms, spreading forwards, may produce symptoms, injuries may cause bruising and there is always the likelihood that a lump may be caused by a hernia. Irritation can be caused when dryness is a problem, depression can incite itching and uncomfortable or over enthusiastic love-making can produce symptoms of many kinds. Oestrogen deficiency can produce a variety of vulvo-vaginitis and very occasionally cancer may develop on or around the vulva. In infants and young girls, by the way, it is worth remembering that the vulva normally look red and although they seem inflamed and infected they are usually quite all right.

Treating vulval problems depends, of course, upon finding the cause. Most mild symptoms can, however, be treated by using a mild saline wash and a simple calamine lotion or cream. In older women, where dryness is a particular problem, an oestrogen cream can work wonders. Antiseptic creams and washes are best avoided since they can produce symptoms and problems of their own.

See also Anatomy (p. 6)

WARTS

They're caused by a virus, they are common, they usually occur in groups or clusters, they're contagious, they're itchy and they can develop into quite huge and unsightly mounds. When they occur on or around the sexual organs they are included in the list of diseases traditionally described as 'venereal'. The incubation period usually lies somewhere between one and nine months.

Although they aren't harmful or dangerous genital warts are often so unacceptable in simple aesthetic terms that their removal is essential. But they should never be removed at home by anyone unskilled. And they certainly shouldn't be attacked with ordinary wart removing ointments or applications. Genital warts can either be removed with diathermy or cryosurgery or they can sometimes be removed by painting with podophyllin paint or ointment. This needs to be done by an expert and it must not be allowed to spread on to healthy skin. It needs to be washed off after eight hours.

If you've got warts on any part of your genitals get professional advice.

See also Sexually transmitted disease (p. 74)

WITHDRAWAL

A form of contraception also known as 'coitus interruptus', 'being careful', 'self control', 'being considerate', 'pulling out', 'getting off at the last but one stop' and so on. Probably best described as both reckless and unnecessarily painful.

The theory is that by taking his penis out of the woman's vagina just before he ejaculates a man can ensure that pregnancy is avoided.

Apart from the fact that this form of so-called contraception isn't much fun for either party the simple fact is that it isn't a very efficient form of contraception.

The problem is caused by the fact that just before ejaculation some sperm are quite likely to leak out of the penis and into the vagina. And there is no way for the man to know that this is happening.

See also Contraception (p. 22)